Getting Started with ResearchKit

Enter the era of medical research using mobile devices with the help of this guide on ResearchKit!

Dhanush Balachandran

Edward Cessna

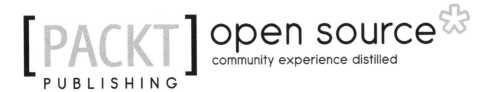

BIRMINGHAM - MUMBAI

Getting Started with ResearchKit

First published: February 2016

Production reference: 1020216

Published by Packt Publishing Ltd.
Livery Place
35 Livery Street
Birmingham B3 2PB, UK.

ISBN 978-1-78588-917-2

www.packtpub.com

Credits

Authors
Dhanush Balachandran
Edward Cessna

Reviewers
Oliver Gepp
Andreas Griesser

Commissioning Editor
Veena Pagare

Acquisition Editor
Kevin Colaco

Content Development Editor
Sumeet Sawant

Technical Editor
Danish Shaikh

Copy Editor
Vibha Shukla

Project Coordinator
Shweta H Birwatkar

Proofreader
Safis Editing

Indexer
Mariammal Chettiyar

Graphics
Disha Haria

Production Coordinator
Nilesh Mohite

Cover Work
Nilesh Mohite

About the Authors

Dhanush Balachandran has a vast experience in creating mobile apps for healthcare industry that include several ResearchKit apps. He was the lead iOS engineer at Jiff, a healthcare start-up and later worked on ResearchKit-based apps for leading institutions. Currently, he is an iOS engineer at DJI. He is also the founder & CEO of mobile app startup, Sortly.

Edward Cessna is the software engineering director for Y Media Labs, a digital agency in Northern California that creates mobile applications. He has three decades of software engineering experience—ranging from embedded software providing cryptographic services to a multitude of iOS applications. He has been working with iOS since its first public release in July 2008. He has managed the development effort for a number of ResearchKit-based applications for leading research institutions.

About the Reviewers

Oliver Gepp is a senior software engineer at Zühlke Group, Switzerland with a strong focus on mobile apps. He has a diploma in media computer science from the Technical University of Dresden, Germany. Most of his projects are in the insurance and banking business, where he covers the whole application life cycle such as business analysis, development, and testing. His passion is developing mobile apps for the iOS platform not only in Swift and Objective-C, but also with cross platform technologies such as Xamarin.

Andreas Griesser is leading the business development at Zühlke Group, Switzerland in the area of LabScience, Pharmaceutical & Biotechnology. He holds a master's degree in telecommunication, mathematics, and informatics from the Technical University of Graz, Austria and a PhD in computer science from the Swiss Federal Institute of Technology, Switzerland (ETH). During his career, he was involved in research projects of real-time three-dimensional scanning, general-purpose computing on graphics processing units (GPGPU), and medical image analysis.

Under his current activities at Zühlke in the healthcare sector, he focuses on topics such as digital transformation and connected devices—not only on a technical level, but also with a business-related perspective.

www.PacktPub.com

Support files, eBooks, discount offers, and more

For support files and downloads related to your book, please visit www.PacktPub.com.

Did you know that Packt offers eBook versions of every book published, with PDF and ePub files available? You can upgrade to the eBook version at www.PacktPub.com and as a print book customer, you are entitled to a discount on the eBook copy. Get in touch with us at service@packtpub.com for more details.

At www.PacktPub.com, you can also read a collection of free technical articles, sign up for a range of free newsletters and receive exclusive discounts and offers on Packt books and eBooks.

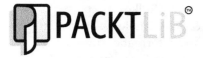

https://www2.packtpub.com/books/subscription/packtlib

Do you need instant solutions to your IT questions? PacktLib is Packt's online digital book library. Here, you can search, access, and read Packt's entire library of books.

Why subscribe?

- Fully searchable across every book published by Packt
- Copy and paste, print, and bookmark content
- On demand and accessible via a web browser

Free access for Packt account holders

If you have an account with Packt at www.PacktPub.com, you can use this to access PacktLib today and view 9 entirely free books. Simply use your login credentials for immediate access.

Table of Contents

Preface

This book helps you get started on creating ResearchKit-based applications. ResearchKit™ is an open source framework introduced by Apple that allows researchers and developers to create powerful apps for medical research.

What this book covers

Chapter 1, *Getting Started*, introduces ResearchKit and explains the anatomy of a ResearchKit-based application.

Chapter 2, *ResearchKit Hello World*, helps you create your first ResearchKit application and teaches how to integrate ResearchKit in your projects.

Chapter 3, *Building Surveys*, covers how to create and present clinical surveys. In this process, you'll also learn about the ResearchKit object model.

Chapter 4, *ResearchKit Informed Consent*, explains how to create, present, and obtain informed consent to participate in clinical studies from the end users.

Chapter 5, *Active Tasks*, covers how to use active tasks—one of the most important features of ResearchKit.

Chapter 6, *Navigable and Custom Tasks*, helps you create smart surveys that can skip questions based on the answers provided by users.

Chapter 7, *Back End Service*, explains how to serialize task results to send to a backend service.

Chapter 8, *Where to go from here*, helps you learn various tools and tips to create real-world ResearchKit applications.

What you need for this book

- iOS Software development tools: Xcode 7.0 or higher
- iOS Device (iPhone or iPad) to use sensors, GPS, and so on
- Basic knowledge of iOS and Swift 2.0

Access to the Internet to download the source code associated with this book

Who this book is for

This book is aimed at medical researchers with basic iOS coding knowledge and iOS developers looking to create clinical research apps.

Conventions

In this book, you will find a number of styles of text that distinguish between different kinds of information. Here are some examples of these styles, and an explanation of their meaning.

Code words in text, database table names, folder names, filenames, file extensions, pathnames, dummy URLs, user input, and Twitter handles are shown as follows: "In `ViewController.swift` file, import ResearchKit framework"

A block of code is set as follows:

```
let step1 = ORKInstructuionStep(identifier:"step1")
step1.title = "Hello World!"
let step2 = ORKInstructuionStep(identifier:"step2")
step2.title = "Bye!"
```

Any command-line input or output is written as follows:

```
git submodule add https://github.com/ResearchKit/ResearchKit.git
```

New terms and **important words** are shown in bold. Words that you see on the screen, in menus or dialog boxes for example, appear in the text like this: "clicking the **Next** button moves you to the next screen".

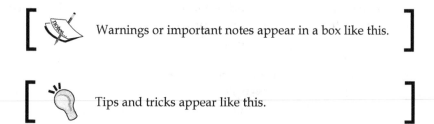

Warnings or important notes appear in a box like this.

Tips and tricks appear like this.

Reader feedback

Feedback from our readers is always welcome. Let us know what you think about this book—what you liked or may have disliked. Reader feedback is important for us to develop titles that you really get the most out of.

To send us general feedback, simply send an e-mail to feedback@packtpub.com, and mention the book title via the subject of your message.

If there is a topic that you have expertise in and you are interested in either writing or contributing to a book, see our author guide on www.packtpub.com/authors.

Customer support

Now that you are the proud owner of a Packt book, we have a number of things to help you to get the most from your purchase.

Downloading the example code

You can download the example code files for all Packt books you have purchased from your account at http://www.packtpub.com. If you purchased this book elsewhere, you can visit http://www.packtpub.com/support and register to have the files e-mailed directly to you.

Errata

Although we have taken every care to ensure the accuracy of our content, mistakes do happen. If you find a mistake in one of our books—maybe a mistake in the text or the code—we would be grateful if you would report this to us. By doing so, you can save other readers from frustration and help us improve subsequent versions of this book. If you find any errata, please report them by visiting http://www.packtpub.com/submit-errata, selecting your book, clicking on the **errata submission form** link, and entering the details of your errata. Once your errata are verified, your submission will be accepted and the errata will be uploaded on our website, or added to any list of existing errata, under the Errata section of that title. Any existing errata can be viewed by selecting your title from http://www.packtpub.com/support.

Piracy

Piracy of copyright material on the Internet is an ongoing problem across all media. At Packt, we take the protection of our copyright and licenses very seriously. If you come across any illegal copies of our works, in any form, on the Internet, please provide us with the location address or website name immediately so that we can pursue a remedy.

Please contact us at copyright@packtpub.com with a link to the suspected pirated material.

We appreciate your help in protecting our authors, and our ability to bring you valuable content.

Questions

You can contact us at questions@packtpub.com if you are having a problem with any aspect of the book, and we will do our best to address it.

1
Getting Started

On March 9, 2015, Apple introduced ResearchKit, a software framework that facilitates the development of health and clinical-based research applications for iOS. Doctors and researchers will be able to collect larger quantities of data frequently and with greater accuracy through the applications built with ResearchKit. The ultimate goal is to increase the research community's knowledge on diseases that could potentially lead to medical breakthroughs in the treatment of the studied diseases.

In conjunction with ResearchKit's announcement, Apple announced and released five ResearchKit-based applications. These applications are as follows:

1. Asthma Health: This is developed by Mount Sinai in order to study asthma triggers and help participants self-manage their asthma. This application makes heavy use of ResearchKit's survey capabilities and custom tasks.

2. mPower: This is developed by the University of Rochester and Sage Bionetworks in order to study the variability in the symptoms of Parkinson's disease. This application utilizes ResearchKit's two-finger tapping, short walk, spatial-span memory, and custom tasks.

3. GlucoSuccess: This is developed by Massachusetts General Hospital to study how diet, physical activity, and medications affect blood glucose levels for participants with type 2 diabetes. This application utilizes ResearchKit's survey capability and custom tasks.

4. Share the Journey: This is developed by the Dana-Farber Cancer Institute, UCLA Fielding School of Public Health, Penn Medicine, and Sage Bionetworks to study the long-term effects of chemotherapy used in the treatment of breast cancer. This application utilizes ResearchKit's survey and custom tasks.

5. MyHeart Counts: This is developed by Stanford Medicine and the University of Oxford in order to study how a participant's lifestyle affects the risk of cardiovascular disease. This application utilizes ResearchKit's fitness-check task and surveys, and custom tasks.

The five initial ResearchKit-based applications shared similar user experience. Using a common application core that's independent of ResearchKit, these applications had a common on-boarding process to enroll new participants in the study, an activity list to present tasks that the researchers wish the participants to carry out, and a dashboard to present the results of the previously carried out tasks. Additionally, these applications used the same backend service to establish accounts, download task schedules and surveys, and upload the collected data in a secure manner.

Apple has open sourced all of the initial ResearchKit applications, and the application core that provides additional services and capabilities beyond these features of ResearchKit.

 Links to the source code, documentation, and other information can be found on www.apple.com/researchkit and www.researchkit.org; the source code is hosted directly on GitHub at https://github.com/researchkit.

The open source applications serve as an example for researchers to undertake the development of their own ResearchKit-based applications. As examples, there are differences between these applications and the ones available from the App Store. In general, copyright material has been removed along with the cryptographic credentials that enable the applications to upload data to the researcher's servers.

What is ResearchKit?

At its core, ResearchKit orchestrates the administering of tasks and recording of the results from each step of the task. ResearchKit's tasks are segregated into modules: surveys, informed consent, and active tasks. Surveys are questionnaires that prompt the participant to answer to a set of questions for the purpose of recording information that can be used for statistical analysis. Surveys support a variety of question types and answer formats. The informed consent module provides the basic mechanism that is necessary to conduct informed consent visually. Active tasks provide the framework that is necessary to allow applications to develop tasks for the participant. On its announcement, ResearchKit was shipped with a number of predefined tasks, as follows:

1. Fitness check: The participant is asked to walk for a specified duration while recording data from various sensors. If the heart-rate data is available at the conclusion of the task, the user is asked to sit down for a duration and the data recording continues.

2. Short Walk: The participant is asked to walk a short distance while data from the accelerometer and pedometer data is being recorded.

3. Audio recording: The participant is asked to record the sound that they make.

4. Finger tapping: The participant is asked to tap two targets on the screen as touch activity and accelerometer data is being recorded.

5. Spatial-span memory: The participant is asked to participate in a game-like task that tests their ability to repeat a pattern of increasing length.

Subsequent chapters will go to greater depths on how to use the predefined activities provided by ResearchKit and construct new active tasks.

Privacy

In a clinical research application, nothing is more important than the privacy of the user's personal information. Whether this information resides in a device or during transmittal to a data-collection server, personal health information must be safeguarded at each step. Information in the device must be protected irrespective of whether the application operating in the foreground, background, or not executing at all. If the information is transmitted to a data-collection server, it must be safeguarded during transmission. Safeguarding data in transit includes protecting the data during transmission as well as ensuring that the data is going to the correct destination.

Safeguarding of personal health information is the responsibility of the application. ResearchKit provides little capability in this regard other than to ensure classes that may contain user information compile with the `NSSecureCoding` protocol. The following security and privacy-related issues must be considered by the application developer:

- The *Data Protection* service is the default level of protection for data files stored in the device by the iOS application.

- The *Data Protection* level for directories that may contain the uploaded data in the background.

- The protection of files containing the data that may be uploaded. The data to be uploaded will need additional levels of protection than those offered by the *Data Protection* service.

- The authentication of the endpoint where data will be uploaded.

Identification, authentication, and authorization

Identification, authentication, and authorization are the key concepts in information security. Identification is simply claiming you are somebody. Authentication is proving that you are who you say you are. Authorization is where an authority gives you the permission to carry out a specific task or set of tasks. It is highly likely that these concepts will come into play for a ResearchKit-based application, considering that the application may record, transmit, and display sensitive information about the participant.

ResearchKit does not provide any support for identification, authentication, or authorization; it is up to the application developer to implement the required functionality. Depending on the requirements of an application, the developer may need to implement features to identify and authenticate a participant for both the iOS device and web services (for example, data collection service). Identifying and authenticating to a device is to ensure that the right person is using the application. Identifying and authenticating to a web service is to ensure that the data is only collected from consented individuals.

For devices with Touch ID, Apple's fingerprint recognition feature, an application developer may use this technology to identify and authenticate a participant to the device. Available in all iOS devices, Apple's keychain technology may be used to store log-on credential for any web services. Once a participant has been authenticated to the device, the application may retrieve the web services' credentials from the keychain.

Informed consent

Informed consent is a standard practice for health providers and clinical researchers in providing health care or conducting clinical research; it is not a concept specific to ResearchKit. Obtaining informed consent from participants, prior to enrolling them in a clinical study, is to ensure that the permission has been given and the participant has a clear understanding of the facts, implications, and consequences of their participation in the study. As such, informed consent and its constituents are a vast topic that is beyond the scope of this book.

ResearchKit provides the mechanism that is necessary to present the informed consent document to the participant as an animated sequence of *pages* as well as the document in its totality. Each page may have *more information* that presents more details on the page's topic. ResearchKit comes with a number of predefined sections, as shown in the following:

- Overview
- Data gathering
- Privacy
- Data use
- Time commitment
- Surveys
- Tasks
- Withdrawal

The informed consent module includes the ability to record the participant's signature if that is required by a study's informed consent process. This is not a digital signature (that is, verifiable and irrevocable) and ResearchKit has no provisions to collect such signatures. It's the application developer's responsibility to provide support for digital signature, if required by the study protocol.

Informed consent is a ResearchKit task. As such, it may be extended in order to comply with the requirements of the study. For example, the consent process for some of the initial ResearchKit applications presents a comprehension quiz that the participants were required to pass in order to be deemed *consented*.

Relationship with HealthKit

Apple promotes HealthKit as a technology that allows iOS applications providing health and fitness services to share data with each other. Effectively, HealthKit is a system-wide, health-specific database with developer services that allow the applications to read and write health data to HealthKit. Given the sensitivity of the data stored in the HealthKit repository, HealthKit will request permission from the user for each requested category of information and whether or not the application is allowed to read or write data of the requested category.

ResearchKit and HealthKit are separate but related technologies. ResearchKit utilizes HealthKit in a variety of ways. ResearchKit tasks may require access to information stored in HealthKit in order to present appropriate feedback to the participant or record such information for statistical analysis. A ResearchKit task may write information to HealthKit (for example, a participant's weight, blood pressure, and so on) after obtaining the participant's permission. Additionally, ResearchKit uses HealthKit to perform unit conversion on the data that is captured from various sensors or read from HealthKit.

Features not provided by ResearchKit

A ResearchKit-based application may need additional features beyond those provided by ResearchKit. The initial set of ResearchKit-based application provide the following capabilities:

- Backend services: In order to be of any use, the recorded data must be transmitted somewhere for analysis. The initial ResearchKit-based applications used a service from a non-profit organization, Sage Bionetworks.

- User feedback of completed tasks: Appropriate levels of feedback to the user create engaging applications that encourages the user to continue using the application. This increases the likelihood of continued data streams from the participants.

- Data security and privacy: Applications must safeguard a participant's personal information by applying the appropriate level data and communication security.

- Passive data collection: Depending on the nature of the research study, it may be beneficial for the application to collect data in the background without direct participant involvement. For example, using location tracking at a low frequency, an application can obtain relative displacements and use it as a measure of socialization.

- Task scheduling: A study may want tasks performed at different frequencies and quantities.

The anatomy of a ResearchKit-based application

The five initial ResearchKit-based applications share a common software architecture. One based on a layered architecture using common software components in order to provide a similar user experience and application functionality. While ResearchKit offers a wealth of opportunities for different types of research applications, the following figure describes a generic architecture that's common to what the initial ResearchKit-based application employed. Using a layered architecture and common components, a developer may create the basis for a family of applications. Such a framework could be used to address the needs for multiple applications at a reduced cost and increased software quality, as shown in the following diagram:

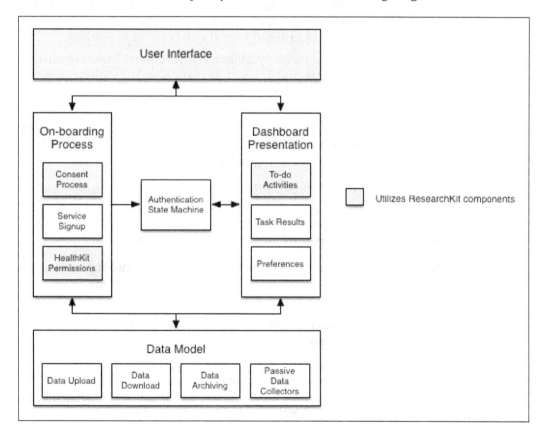

The figure describes a generic architecture that can form the basis of a ResearchKit-based application. Using a layered approach, the architecture has features described in the following paragraphs.

A central Data Model that services the needs for the upper layers and components. This layer includes the following components:

- A *data upload* component that is responsible to upload data, track the success or failure of the upload attempts, retry failed upload attempts, and clean up the data that has been successfully uploaded.

- A *data download* component that either periodically or on-demand, downloads new task schedules, survey contents, and news about the study that the researchers desire to share with participant.

- A *data archiving* component that packages the data to be uploaded to the studies backend server or other destinations. This component can support one or more formats. A key feature of this component is to ensure the confidentiality of the data prior to uploading it to the data collection service. The five initial ResearchKit-based applications used the Cryptographic Message Syntax (RFC 5652) in order to *wrap* the data for safeguarding.

- One or more *passive data collector* components. With the participant's explicit permission, these components could collect the data from the various sensors on the device and then trigger a data upload. For example, in order to determine whether the participants were socializing or homebound, a number of the initial ResearchKit-based applications collected relative displacement of the device location. Relative displacement allows the researchers to determine socialization, while avoiding collecting sensitive location data.

An on-boarding process will be common for ResearchKit-based applications. During this process, the applications could present background information about the study, collect any required demographic information, and perform the consent process (a ResearchKit-based activity). This layer includes the following components:

- A *consent process* component that performs the informed-consent process. ResearchKit supports this activity and provides many features to shape this feature.

- A *service signup* component, if it is necessary for the participant to provide some kind of login credential or identity with a data collection service.

- For applications that retrieve data from HealthKit, a *HealthKit permissions* component could inform the participant in one place as to which data will be collected and why. This would be an excellent place to allow the participant to opt out of the collection for one or more HealthKit parameters.

Given the potential sensitive nature of ResearchKit-based applications, the identity and authentication of the application user as a study participant should always be determined prior to allowing a user to use the application. As a variety of data, events, time triggers, and so on could be input in to the authentication process, this component may best be implemented as a state machine.

Once a user has been authenticated (gone through the on-boarding process and authenticated), the heart of this theoretical application's user interface is the *dashboard*. The *dashboard* layer includes the following components:

- A *to-do activities* component that displays a list of activities that the researchers wish the study participants to accomplish. These activities can include ResearchKit-based tasks (for example, surveys) or custom tasks that do not employ ResearchKit. An example of the latter would be a news component, where the researchers share ongoing information about the study in general.

- A *task results* component, where the application shares the results or summary of the results for completed tasks. If task-aggregated results are available (either baked in the application or downloaded via the *data download* complement), the application could inform the participant how they are performing with respect to the study's population norm.

- A *preference* component that allows the participant to customize the application to serve their need. This would be an excellent place to allow the participant to opt out or opt in to the collection of specific data parameters. Additionally, this component could serve as the vehicle to allow the participants to withdraw from the study.

The top component in this layered architecture is the *user interface* component. This component provides the *heart and soul* from a user's experience point of view. This component will also address any branding requirements levied by the research institution.

Summary

In this chapter, you were introduced to ResearchKit framework and the different aspects of a ResearchKit-based application.

In the next chapter, we will write a simple Hello World ResearchKit-based application.

2
ResearchKit Hello World

In this chapter, we will be creating a simple `Hello World` app using ResearchKit. During this process, you will learn how to integrate ResearchKit in an Xcode project and set up data protection. The second part of the chapter will introduce you to the `Softwareitis` app, which we will be building throughout this book as we study the various aspects of ResearchKit.

Hello World App

Let's get started on building the `Hello World` app.

Create project

Following are the steps to create simple Xcode application:

1. Firstly, note that we will be using Xcode 7 and Swift 2.0 throughout this book and then open Xcode:

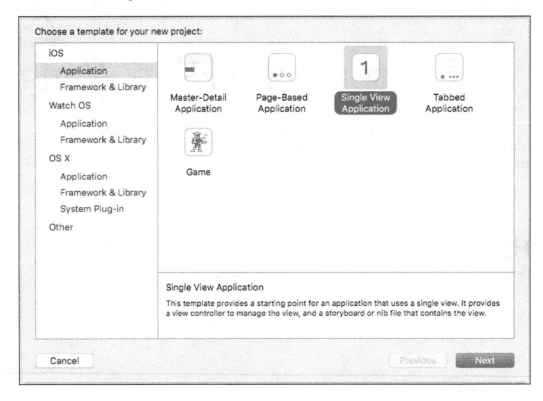

2. Create a new `HelloWorldRK` project as shown in the following image:

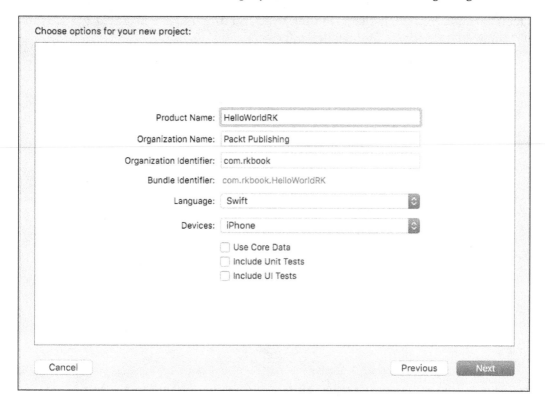

Checkout ResearchKit from GitHub

Open the `terminal` app and `cd` in the `HelloWorldRK` folder, where the
`HelloWorldRK.xcodeproj` file is located. Type the following command to check
ResearchKit from the GitHub repository:

```
git clone https://github.com/ResearchKit/ResearchKit.git ResearchKit
```

> In case you are using Git for version control of your project, it
> is recommended to check ResearchKit as a Git submodule. You
> can use the following command. You can learn more about Git
> submodules at `https://git-scm.com/book/en/v2/Git-`
> `Tools-Submodules`:
>
> ```
> git submodule add https://github.com/ResearchKit/
> ResearchKit.git ResearchKit
> ```

Import ResearchKit

Open the `ResearchKit` folder in **Finder**, drag and drop `ResearchKit.xcodeproj` in `HelloWorldRK` as shown in the following screenshot:

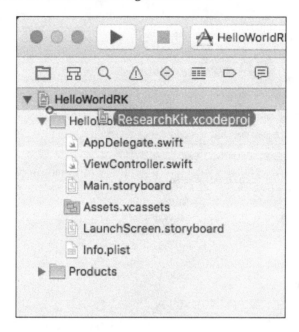

Then, embed the ResearchKit framework by adding it to the **Embedded Binaries** section of the **General** pane for your target as shown in following screenshot:

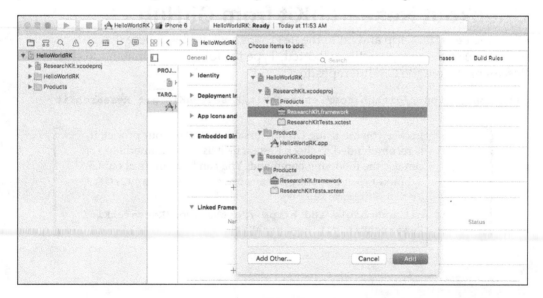

After embedding, the project should appear as shown in the following image:

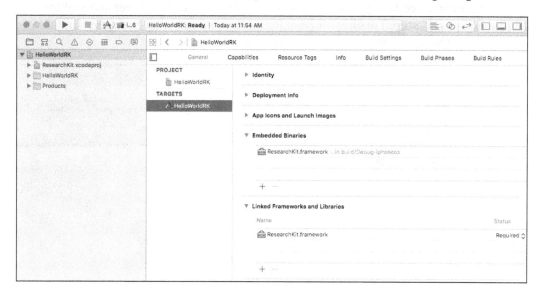

 Build the project (⌘ + B). The absence of build errors indicates successful integration of ResearchKit in the project.

 You can also import ResearchKit in your project using a dependency manager such as CocoaPods or Carthage. Check ResearchKit GitHub page for documentation.

Enable Data Protection

As mentioned in the previous chapter, privacy and data protection are very important for clinical research apps. Therefore, we set up data protection before adding the `Hello World` code.

Enable **Data Protection** in the **Capabilities** section of your target as shown in the following image. Xcode may require you to sign in to your developer account for completion of this step. Turning on Data Protection ensures that the users' folders and files are encrypted and cannot be read while the device is locked.

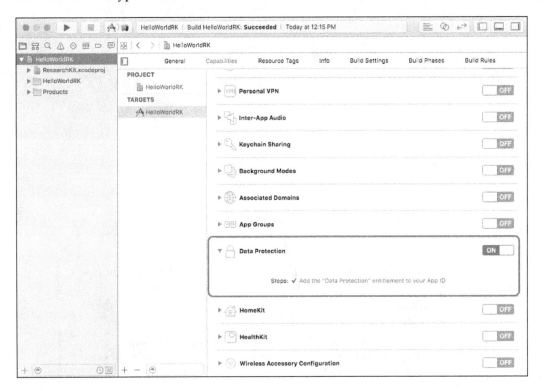

Hello World!

Now, we are ready to show `Hello World` using ResearchKit! This is can be achieved with a few lines of code.

In the `ViewController.swift` file, import ResearchKit framework by adding the following line of code at the top of the file:

```
import ResearchKit
```

Add showHelloWorld method to ViewController class:

```
func showHelloWorld()
{
    //1
    let step1 = ORKInstructionStep(identifier: "step1")
    step1.title = "Hello World!"
```

```
    let step2 = ORKInstructionStep(identifier: "step2")
    step2.title = "Bye!"
    //2
    let task = ORKOrderedTask(identifier: "task", steps: [step1,
step2])
    //3
    let taskViewController = ORKTaskViewController(task: task,
taskRunUUID: nil)
    //4
    taskViewController.delegate = self
    //5
    presentViewController(taskViewController, animated: true,
completion: nil)
}
```

The explanation of the above code is as below:

1. Creates two ORKInstructionStep objects with the step1 and step2 identifiers and sets their title property to Hello World and Bye!. As we will see in the next chapter, ORKInstructionStep displays its title property on the screen.

2. Creates an ORKOrderedTask task object with task identifier and provides two steps in the steps: parameter. The ORKOrderedTask defines an ordered task with a series of steps. We will study more about this in the next chapter.

3. The ORKTaskViewController plays the tasks. This line of code creates an ORKTaskViewController object using the task that we created earlier.

4. Sets the ViewController object as the delegate for the ORKTaskViewController. Xcode will show an error as ViewController does not comply with the ORKTaskViewControllerDelegate protocol yet. We will be fixing this shortly.

5. Presents the task view controller modally using the presentViewController :animated:completion: method of UIViewController.

Add an extension to the ViewController class that complies with the ORKTaskViewControllerDelegate protocol and implements the required taskView Controller:didFinishWithReason:error method, as follows:

```
extension ViewController : ORKTaskViewControllerDelegate
{
    func taskViewController(taskViewController: ORKTaskViewController,
didFinishWithReason reason: ORKTaskViewControllerFinishReason, error:
NSError?)
    {
        //1
```

```
            dismissViewControllerAnimated(true, completion: nil)
        }
    }
```

- `taskViewController:didFinishWithReason:error:` The delegate method is called when task view controller has finished playing the task.
- We invoke the `dismissViewControllerAnimated:completion:` Method of `UIViewController` to dismiss the presented modal view controller.

We will now call `showHelloWorld`. Call the `showHelloWorld` method in the `buttonPressed` action, as follows:

```
    @IBAction func buttonPressed(sender: AnyObject) {
        showHelloWorld()
    }
```

Now, we are ready to run (⌘ + R) the project. You will see the output in the **Simulator** as shown in the following image:

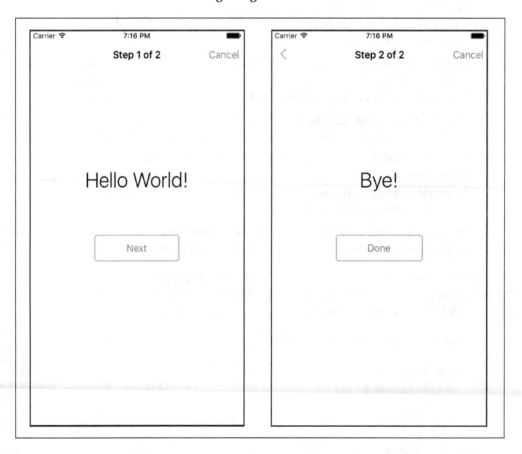

ResearchKit expects steps of a task to have unique identifiers.

 Experiment: Try changing the step2 identifier to step1 and see what Exception do you get.

Introducing Softwareitis

In order to keep it fun and light, we will be developing a clinical research app for a fictitious disease called Softwareitis. This disease is characterized by the constant need to download and try new apps in the smartphone. Throughout this book, we will be building the Softwareitis research app to demonstrate various aspects of ResearchKit.

You can find the Softwareitis.xcodeproj Xcode project in the Chapter_2/ Softwareitis folder of the RKBook GitHub repository. Open it in Xcode and make yourself familiar with this simple app, especially the TableViewController.swift file.

As you can see, the app has just one table view controller with each row of the table view representing a Softwareitis task that a user needs to perform. Currently, it has a demo task, Hello World, which we created in the HelloWorldRK app. Throughout the book, we will be adding new tasks by adding methods to the TableViewController Softwareitis Tasks extension and adding entries to rows in the setupTableViewRows method of TableViewController.swift.

Summary

In this chapter, you learned how to create the Hello World ResearchKit app. You were also introduced to the Softwareitis project, which we will be building for rest of the book.

In the next chapter, let's take a look at creating Surveys at depth and *Introduction to the Basic RK* object model: ORKTask, ORKTaskViewController, and ORKResult.

3
Building Surveys

Surveys are one of the most common tools used in clinical research studies. In this chapter, you will learn how to create, display, and generate results from surveys using ResearchKit. In the process, we will get an overview of the ResearchKit object model. You will also learn how to customize the appearance of the UI elements in ResearchKit.

ResearchKit object model

This section provides a high-level overview of ResearchKit object model using UML-like class diagrams. Understanding the object model will help us utilize the ResearchKit better.

Tasks and steps

Tasks and steps are the fundamental building blocks of ResearchKit. Just like the tasks in real world, the tasks in ResearchKit can be defined with a series of steps. The examples of these tasks can be answering to a five-question survey, a 20 minute cardio activity test, and so on:

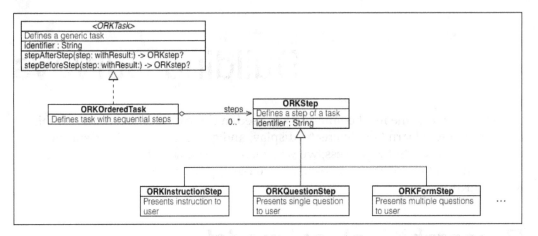

The preceding image shows the object model for tasks and steps. Note that, for the sake of simplicity, the diagram only shows the important properties and methods. Feel free to refer to the ResearchKit API documentation in Xcode for a comprehensive list of properties and methods.

The <ORKTask> is a protocol that defines a generic ResearchKit task. It has a non-nil identifier property to identify the task and two methods: stepBeforeStep and stepAfterStep. The ORKOrderedTask implements these two methods of the <ORKTask> protocol and enables us to represent simple tasks with a fixed order of steps. As you may recall, we used ORKOrderedTask in *Chapter 2, ResearchKit Hello World* to create a Hello World task.

The ORKStep is a base class for a step of a task. ResearchKit provides several subclasses of ORKStep to represent different types of steps. For example, ORKInstructionStep allows us to show instructions or introductory content of a task to the user, ORKQuestionStep is to show a single question, and ORKFormStep is to present a form with multiple questions in a single scrollable page. We will be using these three subclasses in this chapter to create surveys. There are several other subclasses of ORKStep, which we will study in the subsequent chapters.

Task view controller and results

The following diagram shows the object model for the task view controller and results:

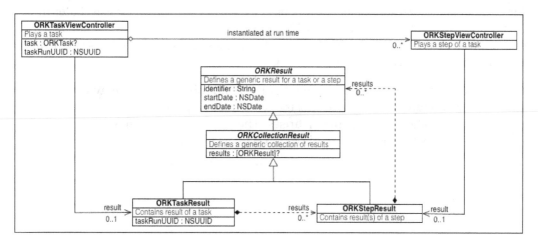

In order to play or execute a task, we instantiate a task object and provide it to ORKTaskViewController. The ORKTaskViewController subclass of UIViewController, *plays* this task by presenting an appropriate ResearchKit framework UI to the user. Internally, ORKTaskViewController instantiates an ORKStepViewController object for each step in order to generate the UI. For the sake of understanding, you can think of the relationship between ORKTaskViewController and ORKStepViewController being similar to that of UINavigationController and UIViewController in the UIKit.

The task property of ORKTaskViewController contains the task that is currently being presented. Whenever a task view controller is presented to the user, a new UUID is created and associated with that presentation or run. This UUID can be read using the taskRunUUID property.

Once a task is presented and successfully completed by the user, the result property of ORKTaskViewController contains the result of the task, which is an instantiation of the ORKTaskResult class. As you can see from the preceding image, ORKTaskResult is a subclass of an abstract ORKCollectionResult class, which in turn is a subclass of the ORKResult base class. The taskRunUUID property of the ORKTaskResult corresponds to the specific run of task view controller. The results property of the ORKTaskResult object contains the results of the steps in the form of the ORKStepResult objects. Similar to ORKTaskResult, ORKStepResult is also a subclass of ORKCollectionResult.

The `results` property of the `ORKStepResult` object contains one or more results of an individual step. This could be an answer to a question that is presented in a question step or an array of answers for a form step. Each result is represented in the form of an `ORKResult` object or an object of its specialized subclasses. Later in this chapter (as well as rest of the book), we will come across several `ORKResult` subclasses. For the sake of clarity and simplicity, these subclasses of `ORKResult` are not shown in the preceding image.

Pay special attention to the arrangement of the result objects as this may later cause confusion when trying to access the results for steps. Feel free to revisit these diagrams when such confusion arises. The following diagram shows the arrangement of `ORKTaskResult` and `ORKStepResult` from a different perspective:

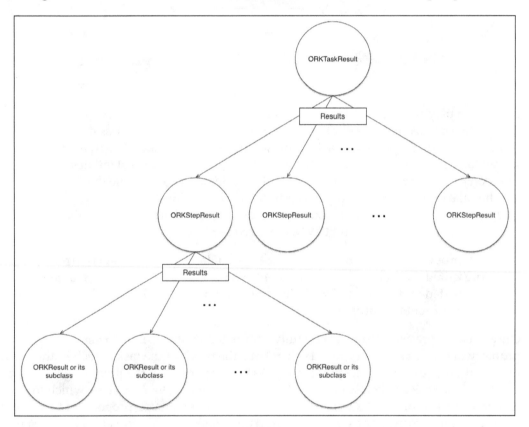

Building surveys

Now that you have learned about the results of tasks from the previous section, we can modify the `Softwareitis` project to incorporate processing of the task results. In the `TableViewController.swift` file, let's update the `rows` data structure to include the reference for `processResultsMethod:` as shown in the following:

```
//Array of dictionaries. Each dictionary contains [ rowTitle :
(didSelectRowMethod, processResultsMethod) ]
var rows : [ [String : ( didSelectRowMethod:()->(), processResultsMeth
od:(ORKTaskResult?)->()   )] ] = []
```

Update the `ORKTaskViewControllerDelegate` method `taskViewController(taskViewController:, didFinishWithReason:, error:)` in `TableViewController` to call `processResultsMethod`, as shown in the following:

```
func taskViewController(taskViewController: ORKTaskViewController,
didFinishWithReason reason: ORKTaskViewControllerFinishReason, error:
NSError?)
{
    if let indexPath = tappedIndexPath
    {
        //1
        let rowDict = rows[indexPath.row]
        if let tuple = rowDict.values.first
        {
            //2
            tuple.processResultsMethod(taskViewController.result)
        }
    }
    dismissViewControllerAnimated(true, completion: nil)
}
```

1. Retrieves the dictionary of the tapped row and its associated tuple containing the `didSelectRowMethod` and `processResultsMethod` references from `rows`.

2. Invokes the `processResultsMethod` with `taskViewController.result` as the parameter.

Now, we are ready to create our first survey. In `Survey.swift`, under the `Surveys` folder, you will find two methods defined in the `TableViewController` extension: `showSurvey()` and `processSurveyResults()`. These are the methods that we will be using to create the survey and process the results.

Instruction step

The instruction step is used to show instruction or introductory content to the user at the beginning or middle of a task. It does not produce any result as it's an informational step. We can create an instruction step using the ORKInstructionStep object. It has title and detailText properties to set the appropriate content. It also has the image property to show an image.

The ORKCompletionStep is a special type of ORKInstructionStep used to show the completion of a task. The ORKCompletionStep shows an animation to indicate the completion of the task along with title and detailText, similar to ORKInstructionStep.

In creating our first Softwareitis survey, let's use the following two steps to show the information:

```
func showSurvey()
{
    //1
    let instStep = ORKInstructionStep(identifier: "Instruction Step")
    instStep.title = "Softwareitis Survey"
    instStep.detailText = "This survey demonstrates different question types."
    //2
    let completionStep = ORKCompletionStep(identifier: "Completion Step")
    completionStep.title = "Thank you for taking this survey!"
    //3
    let task = ORKOrderedTask(identifier: "first survey", steps: [instStep, completionStep])
    //4
    let taskViewController = ORKTaskViewController(task: task, taskRunUUID: nil)
    taskViewController.delegate = self
    presentViewController(taskViewController, animated: true, completion: nil)
}
```

The explanation of the preceding code is as follows:

1. Creates an ORKInstructionStep object with an identifier "Instruction Step" and sets its title and detailText properties.

2. Creates an ORKCompletionStep object with an identifier "Completion Step" and sets its title property.

3. Creates an `ORKOrderedTask` object with the `instruction` and `completion` step as its parameters.

4. Creates an `ORKTaskViewController` object with the ordered task that was previously created and presents it to the user.

Let's update the `processSurveyResults` method to process the results of the instruction step and the completion step as shown in the following:

```
func processSurveyResults(taskResult: ORKTaskResult?)
{
    if let taskResultValue = taskResult
    {
        //1
        print("Task Run UUID : " + taskResultValue.taskRunUUID.
UUIDString)
        print("Survey started at : \(taskResultValue.startDate!)
Ended at : \(taskResultValue.endDate!)")
        //2
        if let instStepResult = taskResultValue.
stepResultForStepIdentifier("Instruction Step")
        {
            print("Instruction Step started at : \(instStepResult.
startDate!)   Ended at : \(instStepResult.endDate!)")
        }
        //3
        if let compStepResult = taskResultValue.
stepResultForStepIdentifier("Completion Step")
        {
            print("Completion Step started at : \(compStepResult.
startDate!)   Ended at : \(compStepResult.endDate!)")
        }
    }
}
```

The explanation of the preceding code is given in the following:

1. As mentioned at the beginning of this chapter, each task run is associated with a UUID. This UUID is available in the `taskRunUUID` property, which is printed in the first line. The second line prints the start and end date of the task. These are useful user analytics data with regards to how much time the user took to finish the survey.

2. Obtains the ORKStepResult object corresponding to the instruction step using the stepResultForStepIdentifier method of the ORKTaskResult object. Prints the start and end date of the step result, which shows the amount of time for which the instruction step was shown before the user pressed the **Get Started** or **Cancel** buttons. Note that, as mentioned earlier, ORKInstructionStep does not produce any results. Therefore, the results property of the ORKStepResult object will be nil. You can use a breakpoint to stop the execution at this line of code and verify it.

3. Obtains the ORKStepResult object corresponding to the completion step. Similar to the instruction step, this prints the start and end date of the step.

The preceding code produces screens as shown in the following image:

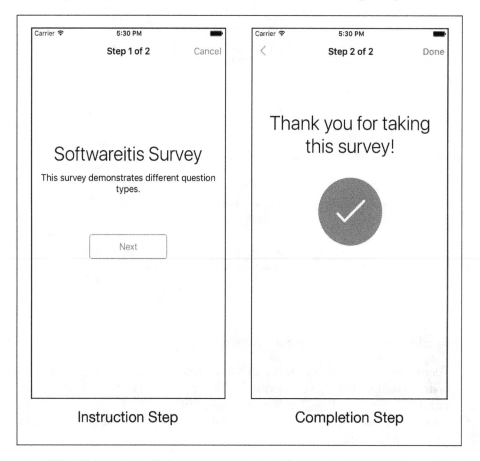

After the **Done** button is pressed in the completion step, Xcode prints the output that is similar to the following:

```
Task Run UUID : 0A343E5A-A5CD-4E7C-88C6-893E2B10E7F7
Survey started at : 2015-08-11 00:41:03 +0000    Ended at : 2015-08-
11 00:41:07 +0000

Instruction Step started at : 2015-08-11 00:41:03 +0000    Ended at :
2015-08-11 00:41:05 +0000

Completion Step started at : 2015-08-11 00:41:05 +0000    Ended at :
2015-08-11 00:41:07 +0000
```

Question step

The question steps make up the body of a survey. ResearchKit supports question steps with various answer types such as boolean (Yes or No), numeric input, date selection, and so on.

Let's first create a question step with the simplest boolean answer type by inserting the following line of code in showSurvey():

```
let question1 = ORKQuestionStep(identifier: "question 1",
title: "Have you ever been diagnosed with Softwareitis?", answer:
ORKAnswerFormat.booleanAnswerFormat())
```

The preceding code creates an ORKQuestionStep object with identifier: "question1", title with the question, and an ORKBooleanAnswerFormat object created using the booleanAnswerFormat() class method of ORKAnswerFormat. The answer type for a question is determined by the type of the ORKAnswerFormat object that is passed in the answer parameter. The ORKAnswerFormat has several subclasses such as ORKBooleanAnswerFormat, ORKNumericAnswerFormat, and so on. Here, we are using ORKBooleanAnswerFormat.

Don't forget to insert the created question step in the ORKOrderedTask steps parameter by updating the following line:

```
let task = ORKOrderedTask(identifier: "first survey", steps:
[instStep, question1, completionStep])
```

When you run the preceding changes in Xcode and start the survey, you will see the question step with the Yes or No options. We have now successfully added a boolean question step to our survey, as shown in the following image:

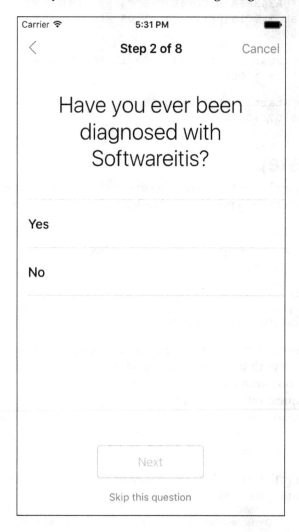

Now, its time to process the results of this question step. The result is produced in an ORKBooleanQuestionResult object. Insert the following lines of code in processSurveyResults():

```
//1
if let question1Result = taskResultValue.stepResultForStepIdentifier
("question 1")?.results?.first as? ORKBooleanQuestionResult
{
    //2
```

```
    if question1Result.booleanAnswer != nil
    {
        let answerString = question1Result.booleanAnswer!.boolValue ?
"Yes" : "No"
        print("Answer to question 1 is \(answerString)")
    }
    else
    {
        print("question 1 was skipped")
    }
}
```

The explanation of the preceding code is as follows:

1. Obtains the ORKBooleanQuestionResult object by first obtaining the step result using the stepResultForStepIdentifier method, accessing its results property, and finally obtaining the only ORKBooleanQuestionResult object available in the results array.

2. The booleanAnswer property of ORKBooleanQuestionResult contains the user's answer. We will print the answer if booleanAnswer is non-nil. If booleanAnswer is nil, it indicates that the user has skipped answering the question by pressing the **Skip this question** button.

 You can disable the skipping-of-a-question step by setting its optional property to false.

We can add the numeric and scale type question steps using the following lines of code in showSurvey():

```
//1
let question2 = ORKQuestionStep(identifier: "question 2", title:
"How many apps do you download per week?", answer: ORKAnswerFormat.
integerAnswerFormatWithUnit("Apps per week"))
//2
let answerFormat3 = ORKNumericAnswerFormat.
scaleAnswerFormatWithMaximumValue(10, minimumValue: 0, defaultValue:
5, step: 1, vertical: false, maximumValueDescription: nil,
minimumValueDescription: nil)
let question3 = ORKQuestionStep(identifier: "question 3",
title: "How many apps do you download per week (range)?", answer:
answerFormat3)
```

The explanation of the preceding code is as follows:

1. Creates ORKQuestionStep with the ORKNumericAnswerFormat object, created using the integerAnswerFormatWithUnit method with Apps per week as the unit. Feel free to refer to the ORKNumericAnswerFormat documentation for decimal answer format and other validation options that you can use.

2. First creates ORKScaleAnswerFormat with minimum and maximum values and step. Note that the number of step increments required to go from minimumValue to maximumValue cannot exceed 10. For example, maximum value of 100 and minimum value of 0 with a step of 1 is not valid and ResearchKit will raise an exception. The step needs to be at least 10. In the second line, ORKScaleAnswerFormat is fed in the ORKQuestionStep object.

The following lines in processSurveyResults() process the results from the number and the scale questions:

```
//1
if let question2Result = taskResultValue.stepResultForStepIdentifier
("question 2")?.results?.first as? ORKNumericQuestionResult
{
    if question2Result.numericAnswer != nil
    {
        print("Answer to question 2 is \(question2Result.
numericAnswer!)")
    }
    else
    {
        print("question 2 was skipped")
    }
}
//2
if let question3Result = taskResultValue.stepResultForStepIdentifier
("question 3")?.results?.first as? ORKScaleQuestionResult
{
    if question3Result.scaleAnswer != nil
    {
        print("Answer to question 3 is \(question3Result.
scaleAnswer!)")
    }
    else
    {
        print("question 3 was skipped")
    }
}
```

The explanation of the preceding code is as follows:

1. The question step with ORKNumericAnswerFormat generates the result with the ORKNumericQuestionResult object. The numericAnswer property of ORKNumericQuestionResult contains the answer value if the question is not skipped by the user.

2. The scaleAnswer property of ORKScaleQuestionResult contains the answer for a scale question.

As you can see in the following image, the numeric type question generates a free form text field to enter the value, while scale type generates a slider:

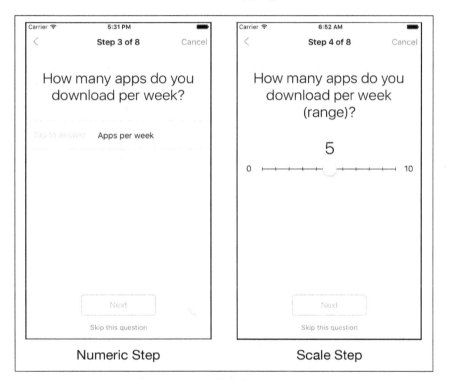

Let's look at a slightly complicated question type with ORKTextChoiceAnswerFormat. In order to use this answer format, we need to create the ORKTextChoice objects beforehand. Each text choice object provides the necessary data to act as a choice in a single choice or multiple choice question. The following lines in showSurvey() create a single choice question with three options:

```
//1
let textChoice1 = ORKTextChoice(text: "Games", detailText: nil,
value: 1, exclusive: false)
```

```
   let textChoice2 = ORKTextChoice(text: "Lifestyle", detailText: nil,
value: 2, exclusive: false)
   let textChoice3 = ORKTextChoice(text: "Utility", detailText: nil,
value: 3, exclusive: false)
   //2
   let answerFormat4 = ORKNumericAnswerFormat.
choiceAnswerFormatWithStyle(ORKChoiceAnswerStyle.SingleChoice,
textChoices: [textChoice1, textChoice2, textChoice3])
   let question4 = ORKQuestionStep(identifier: "question 4",
title: "Which category of apps do you download the most?", answer:
answerFormat4)
```

The explanation of the preceding code is as follows:

1. Creates text choice objects with `text` and `value`. When a choice is selected, the object in the `value` property is returned in the corresponding `ORKChoiceQuestionResult` object. The `exclusive` property is used in multiple choice questions context. Refer to the documentation for its use.

2. First, creates an `ORKChoiceAnswerFormat` object with the text choices that were previously created and specifies a single choice type using the `ORKChoiceAnswerStyle` enum. You can easily change this question to multiple choice question by changing the `ORKChoiceAnswerStyle` enum to multiple choice. Then, an `ORKQuestionStep` object is created using the answer format object.

Processing the results from a single or multiple choice question is shown in the following. Needless to say, this code goes in the `processSurveyResults()` method:

```
   //1
   if let question4Result = taskResultValue.stepResultForStepIdentifier
("question 4")?.results?.first as? ORKChoiceQuestionResult
   {
       //2
       if question4Result.choiceAnswers != nil
       {
           print("Answer to question 4 is \(question4Result.
choiceAnswers!)")
       }
       else
       {
           print("question 4 was skipped")
       }
   }
```

The explanation of the preceding code is as follows:

1. The result for a single or multiple choice question is returned in an `ORKChoiceQuestionResult` object.
2. The `choiceAnswers` property holds the array of values for the chosen options.

The following image shows the generated choice question UI for the preceding code:

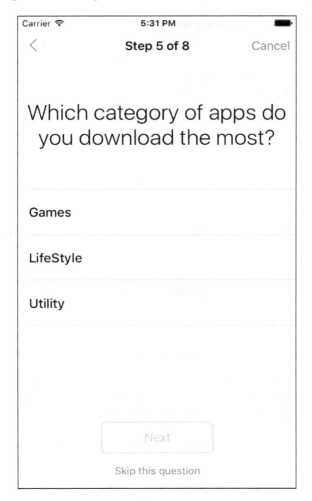

There are several other question types, which operate in a very similar manner like the ones we discussed so far. You can find them in the documentations of `ORKAnswerFormat` and `ORKResult` classes. The `Softwareitis` project has implementation of two additional types: date format and time interval format.

Using custom tasks, you can create surveys that can skip the display of certain questions based on the answers that the users have provided so far. For example, in a smoking habits survey, if the user chooses the "I do not smoke" option, then there is the ability to not display the "How many cigarettes per day?" question.

Form step

A form step allows you to combine several related questions in a single scrollable page and reduces the number of the **Next** button taps for the user. The ORKFormStep object is used to create the form step. The questions in the form are represented using the ORKFormItem objects. The ORKFormItem is similar to ORKQuestionStep, in which it takes the same parameters (title and answer format).

Let's create a new survey with a form step by creating a form.swift extension file and adding the form entry to the rows array in TableViewController.swift, as shown in the following:

```
func setupTableViewRows()
{
    rows += [
        ["Survey" : (didSelectRowMethod: self.showSurvey,
processResultsMethod: self.processSurveyResults)],
        //1
        ["Form" : (didSelectRowMethod: self.showForm,
processResultsMethod: self.processFormResults)]
            ]
}
```

The explanation of the preceding code is as follows:

1. The "Form" entry is added to the rows array to create a new form survey with the showForm() method to show the form survey and the processFormResults() method to process the results from the form.

The following code shows the showForm() method in the Form.swift file:

```
func showForm()
{
    //1
    let instStep = ORKInstructionStep(identifier: "Instruction Step")
    instStep.title = "Softwareitis Form Type Survey"
    instStep.detailText = "This survey demonstrates a form type step."
    //2
```

```
    let question1 = ORKFormItem(identifier: "question 1", text:
"Have you ever been diagnosed with Softwareitis?", answerFormat:
ORKAnswerFormat.booleanAnswerFormat())
    let question2 = ORKFormItem(identifier: "question 2", text:
"How many apps do you download per week?", answerFormat:
ORKAnswerFormat.integerAnswerFormatWithUnit("Apps per week"))
    //3
    let formStep = ORKFormStep(identifier: "form step", title:
"Softwareitis Survey", text: nil)
    formStep.formItems = [question1, question2]
    //1
    let completionStep = ORKCompletionStep(identifier: "Completion
Step")
    completionStep.title = "Thank you for taking this survey!"
    //4
    let task = ORKOrderedTask(identifier: "survey with form", steps:
[instStep, formStep, completionStep])
    let taskViewController = ORKTaskViewController(task: task,
taskRunUUID: nil)
    taskViewController.delegate = self
    presentViewController(taskViewController, animated: true,
completion: nil)
}
```

The explanation of the preceding code is as follows:

1. Creates an instruction and a completion step, similar to the earlier survey.

2. Creates two `ORKFormItem` objects using the questions from the earlier survey. Notice the similarity with the `ORKQuestionStep` constructors.

3. Creates the `ORKFormStep` object with an `identifier` form step and sets the `formItems` property of the `ORKFormStep` object with the `ORKFormItem` objects that are created earlier.

4. Creates an ordered task using the instruction, form, and completion steps and presents it to the user using a new `ORKTaskViewController` object.

The results are processed using the following `processFormResults()` method:

```
func processFormResults(taskResult: ORKTaskResult?)
{
    if let taskResultValue = taskResult
    {
        //1
        if let formStepResult = taskResultValue.
stepResultForStepIdentifier("form step"), formItemResults =
formStepResult.results
```

```
                {
                    //2
                    for result in formItemResults
                    {
                        //3
                        switch result
                        {
                        case let booleanResult as ORKBooleanQuestionResult:
                            if booleanResult.booleanAnswer != nil
                            {
                                let answerString = booleanResult.
booleanAnswer!.boolValue ? "Yes" : "No"
                                print("Answer to \(booleanResult.identifier)
is \(answerString)")
                            }
                            else
                            {
                                print("\(booleanResult.identifier) was
skipped")
                            }
                        case let numericResult as ORKNumericQuestionResult:
                            if numericResult.numericAnswer != nil
                            {
                                print("Answer to \(numericResult.identifier)
is \(numericResult.numericAnswer!)")
                            }
                            else
                            {
                                print("\(numericResult.identifier) was
skipped")
                            }
                        default: break
                        }
                    }
                }
            }
        }
    }
```

The explanation of the preceding code is as follows:

1. Obtains the `ORKStepResult` object of the form step and unwraps the form item results from the `results` property.

2. Iterates through each of the `formItemResults`, each of which will be the result for a question in the form.

3. The `switch` statement detects the different types of question results and accesses the appropriate property that contains the answer.

The following image shows the form step:

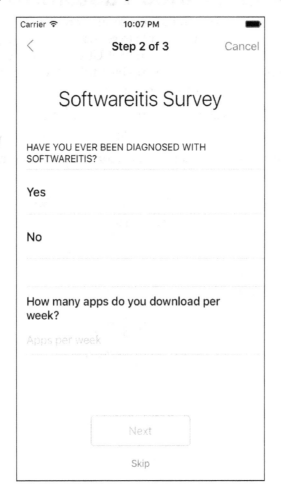

Considerations for real-world surveys

Many clinical research studies that are conducted using a pen and paper tend to have well established surveys. When you try to convert these surveys to ResearchKit, they may not convert perfectly. Some questions and answer choices may have to be reworded so that they can fit on a phone screen. You are advised to work closely with the clinical researchers so that the changes in the surveys still produce comparable results with their pen and paper counterparts. Another aspect to consider is to eliminate some of the survey questions if the answers can be found elsewhere in the user's device. For example, age, blood type, and so on, can be obtained from HealthKit if the user has already set them. This will help in improving the user experience of your app.

BONUS: Appearance customization

ResearchKit honors the values set in the appearance proxies. Therefore, you can use the `appearance` method of UI elements to set its `appearance` properties and their appearance will be changed in ResearchKit UI as well. For example, you can update the tint color throughout the app by adding the following line in the `application(application: didFinishLaunchingWithOptions:)` method:

```
UIView.appearance().tintColor = UIColor(red: 0xA7/0xFF, green:
0x57/0xFF, blue: 0x9D/0xFF, alpha: 1.0)
```

The following image shows the updated tint color of the buttons in the instruction step:

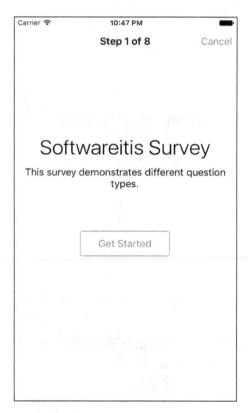

Summary

In this chapter, you learned how to create Surveys using ResearchKit.

In the next chapter, let's study how to obtain informed consent from the users before enrolling them to participate in a clinical research study.

4

ResearchKit Informed Consent

Informed consent is a vital step for clinical research studies. ResearchKit provides a flexible framework to present and obtain informed consent and produce the informed consent document. This framework is based on ResearchKit's tasks, steps, and view controllers. The application developer has the freedom and flexibility to add custom steps in order to address the study-specific steps in its consent process.

All five of the initial ResearchKit-based applications obtained informed consent during the on-boarding process. Even though these applications were based on a common code base, each application had their unique steps in the consent process. For example, the *mPower* and *Share the Journey* applications required the participant to take and pass a comprehension quiz. Similarly, the *Asthma* application also required a comprehension quiz; however, it presented the quiz in a different manner.

The four principal ResearchKit features that facilitate informed consent are as follows:

- Consent document: This contains the content for the informed consent process
- Visual consent step: This presents the consent content in a more consumable manner
- Consent review step: This presents the consent document and elicits consent from the user
- Consent sharing step: This asks the participant how widely they wish to share their data

Consent document

The ORKConsentDocument class is the heart of the informed consent process; it is the container of the information that is to be presented to the participant. This class drives the visual consent step (ORKVisualConsentStep), consent review step (ORKConsentReviewStep), and production of the informed consent document in a PDF. Consent documents have a title and the signature page of the document has a title and page content property; consent documents may have or require one or more signatures.

The properties and relationships of ORKConsentDocument are depicted in the following diagram:

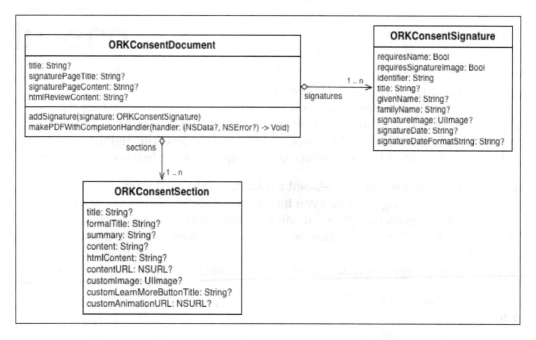

Creating a consent document and setting its properties are accomplished simply by the following:

```
// 1
let document = ORKConsentDocument()
// 2
document.title = "Example Consent"
document.signaturePageTitle = "Consent"
document.signaturePageContent = "I agree to participate in this
research study."
```

Instantiate ORKConsentDocument using the default initializer.

Set the consent document properties. In the production application, strings assigned to ResearchKit properties should be localized.

Instances of `ORKConsentDocument` may have one or more signatures attached to the document. These signatures are represented with instances of `ORKConsentSignature` and are attached to a document via the `addSignature` method on `ORKConsentDocument`. Signature objects have a number of optional attributes: `title`, `givenName`, `familyName`, `signatureImage`, `signatureDate`, and `signatureDateFormatString`. The optional nature of the name and the signature image attributes are controlled by the `requiresName` and `requiresSignatureImage` properties.

Constructing a signature object for the participant, setting its title, and assigning it to a document is accomplished by the following:

```
// 1
let signature = ORKConsentSignature(forPersonWithTitle: "Participant",
    dateFormatString: nil,
    identifier: "ParticipantSignature")
    consentDocument.addSignature(signature)
```

The signature identifier (`ParticipantSignature`, in this example) can be used to find or replace a signature in an `ORKConsentDocument` object. These identifiers may also be used to identify a signature in the results of the `ORKConsentReviewStep`, which are to be discussed in the following.

Adding a signature object for the investigator is accomplished similarly, as shown in the following:

```
// 1
let signatureImage = UIImage(named: "signature")!
// 2
let signature = ORKConsentSignature(forPersonWithTitle:
"Investigator",
                    dateFormatString: nil,
                    identifier: "InvestigatorSignature",
                    givenName: "John",
                    familyName: "Smith",
                    signatureImage: signatureImage,
                    dateString: "3/9/15")
consentDocument.addSignature(investigatorSignature)
```

These steps are explained in the following:

Load an image of the investigator's signature from a `signature` file. This code snippet assumes the image file is in the application bundle. The signature object is created using a different initializer method from the previous example. It represents the investigator's signature that is previously captured at the indicated date.

Similar to the paper-based consent documents, instances of `ORKConsentDocument` are broken down to multiple sections. These sections are represented with instances of `ORKConsentSection`. On release, ResearchKit supported the following section types:

- `Overview`: This provides an overview of the informed consent process.
- `DataGathering`: This informs the user that sensor data will be collected.
- `Privacy`: This provides a description of the study's privacy policies.
- `DataUse`: This describes how the collected data will be used by the study.
- `TimeCommitment`: This describes how much time will be required from the participant.
- `StudySurvey`: This describes the surveys used in the study and how the collected data will be used.
- `StudyTasks`: This describes the active tasks used in the study, the purpose of the tasks, and any associated risk.
- `Withdrawing`: This describes how the participant withdraws from the study and the study's policies regarding the collected data.
- `Custom`: Custom sections do not have a predefined title, summary, content, image, or animation. Consent documents may have zero or more custom sections, as required.
- `OnlyInDocument`: This is a custom section that is not presented during the visual consent step.

Instances of `ORKConsentSection` are assigned to a document by simply assigning an array of sections to the sections property on the `ORKConsentDocument` class. The order of the sections in the `sections` property is the order in which relevant information appears in the visual consent and consent review step.

The content for a consent section may be specified in different ways, depending on the requirements of the application. This information is displayed when the user taps the **Learn More** button and appears in the consent document itself. The developer's options to specify the content are as follows:

- The `content` property: Plain text content
- The `htmlContent` property: Formatted content using HTML
- The `contentURL` property: URL to a UIWebView-loadable document

One or all of these options may be specified; however, only one will be used. The content property has the lowest precedence of these three properties and is used only if htmlContent and contentURL are nil. The value for htmlContent will be used if it is non-nil and contentURL is nil. The contentURL property overrides the other two content properties if it is non-nil.

Creating sections for the informed consent document is accomplished as follows:

```
// 1
let overview = ORKConsentSection(type: .Overview)
overview.summary = "Summary Text"
overview.htmlContent = "<ul><li>Lorem</li><li>ipsum</li></
ul><p>Consent Information</p>"
// 2
let custom = ORKConsentSection(type: .Custom)
custom.title = "Example Custom Section"
custom.summary = "Custom Summary Text"
custom.content = "Custom Section Content"
document.sections = [overview, custom]
```

The explanation of the code is as follows:

1. Create an overview section (ORKConsentSectionType.Overview) using the predefined *overview* consent section. Predefined consent sections have default localized titles and **Learn More** button titles. Applications will need to provide the summary line and actual Learn More content.

2. Create a custom consent section using the ORKConsentSectionType.Custom type. The custom consent sections must provide a title, summary, content, and a title for the **Learn More** button.

The consent document drives the visual consent and consent review step. By default, the informed consent document is the concatenation of the content from each section along with the signature page. If there's a need for the informed consent document to be of a specific format that differs from the content of the consent sections, ResearchKit allows the document for the informed consent review to be separately specified using the htmlReviewContent property.

Visual consent step

ResearchKit provides functionality to visually present the informed consent document. When an instance of ORKVisualConsentStep is included as a step of a ResearchKit task, the sections of the consent document are presented as an animated sequence of pages. Each displayed page contains the following information:

- **Title**: This is the section title displayed at the top of the page. The text for the title comes from the title property.

- **Short Summary**: A short summary of the section displayed under the section title. The text for the summary comes from the summary property.

- **Learn More button**: When tapped by the user, this button triggers the modal display of the section's content.

- **Image**: A section-relevant image, displayed above the section title.

- **Animation**: This is the transition animation from the image on one section to the image on the subsequent section.

The **Learn More** button is only displayed if there is content information assigned to the section; a non-nil value must be assigned to either the content, htmlContent, or contentURL property. The text displayed in the **Learn More** button may be changed via the customLearnMoreButtonTitle property in the section.

In order to be usable by ORKVisualConsentStep, the consent document must have at least one consent section that is not of the ORKConsentSectionTypeOnlyInDocument type. With a proper consent document, creating a task that presents the visual consent is accomplished as follows:

```
// 1
let document = consentDocument()
// 2
let visualConsentStep = ORKVisualConsentStep(identifier:
"VisualConsentStep", document: document)
// 3
let task = ORKOrderedTask(identifier: "ConsentTask", steps:
[visualConsentStep])
let taskViewController = ORKTaskViewController(task: task,
taskRunUUID: nil)
taskViewController.delegate = self
presentViewController(taskViewController, animated: true, completion:
nil)
```

The explanation of the code is as follows:

1. The consent document object (an instance of ORKConsentDocument) is created by the non-ResearchKit consentDocument function.

2. Creates the visual consent step by instantiating the ORKVisualConsentStep class passing in the consent document object.

3. The ORKOrderedTask is a ResearchKit task that, in this case, carries out the single *visual consent* step. Presenting the task and, hence, the individual steps is orchestrated by the task view controller.

Consent review step

The ORKConsentReviewStep is used to initiate the consent review process. This process is where the user reviews the informed consent document and provides their name and signature. The steps of this process are as follows:

1. **Consent document review step**: The consent document is displayed for the participant to review. The participant must explicitly agree to the consent document and confirm their agreement before they can proceed to the next step.

2. **Recording participant name step**: The participants are asked to enter their first (given) and last (family) name. Recording the participant's name may be an optional step.

3. **Recording signature step**: The participant is asked for their signature by presenting a signature line where the participant may draw their signature. Recording the participant's signature may be an optional step.

The content for the consent review process comes from the consent document (instance of ORKConsentDocument) provided to the ORKConsentReviewStep object. This content is generated in one of the following two ways:

1. As a concatenation of the consent sections in the consent document object. This information can come from either the content, htmlContent, or contentURL property.

2. The htmlReviewContent document property contains an HTML string that renders the document.

Whether the consent review process records the participant's name and signature is up to the developer. If the requiresName property on the ORKConsentSignature instance is set to false, then ResearchKit will not attempt to collect the participant's name. Similarly, if the requiresSignatureImage property on the ORKConsentSignature instance is set to false, then the participant's signature will not be requested.

Setting up the consent review step is similar to setting up the visual consent step, as shown in the following:

```
//  1
let document = consentDocument()
//  2
let signature = document.signatures!.first
signature!.requiresName = false
//  3
//  Note: to prevent the app from asking for the participant's
signature, pass nil for the `signature` parameter.
let reviewConsentStep = ORKConsentReviewStep(identifier:
"ConsentReviewStep",
        signature: signature,
        inDocument: document)
//  4
reviewConsentStep.reasonForConsent = "zz Lorem ipsum dolor sit amet."
//  5
let task = ORKOrderedTask(identifier: "ConsentTask", steps:
[reviewConsentStep])
//  6
let taskViewController = ORKTaskViewController(task: task,
taskRunUUID: nil)
taskViewController.delegate = self
presentViewController(taskViewController, animated: true, completion:
nil)
```

The explanation for the preceding code is as follows:

1. The consent document object (an instance of ORKConsentDocument) is created by the non-ResearchKit function, consentDocument.

2. The first signature added to the consent document in the consentDocument function is the participant's signature.

3. Create the consent review step by instantiating an instance of ORKConsentReviewStep passing in the consent document and the participant's signature object.

4. The reasonForConsent property is the text in the alert presented to the user when the application explicitly elicits the user's consent.

5. For demonstration purposes, create a ResearchKit task consisting of the single reviewConsentStep step.

6. Instantiate a ResearchKit task view controller passing in the task created in the fifth step.

7. This view controller will present the following:

   ° Present the consent document: This is a concatenation of the content from all consent sections in the consent document object. This view has the **Disagree** and **Agree** buttons.

   ° If the user taps the **Agree** button, this view controller presents a modal alert consisting of the `reasonForConsent` and the **Cancel** and **Agree** buttons. The participant must tap the **Agree** button in order to be consented.

Consent sharing

The five initial ResearchKit-based applications included a data-sharing step during their on-boarding process. Through the use of the `ORKConsentSharingStep` class, these applications asked the participants how widely they wished to share their data. Instances of `ORKConsentSharingStep` presented the following two options:

1. Share collected data with the study institution and qualified researchers worldwide.

2. Only share collected data with the study institution and its partner.

The `ORKConsentSharingStep` class is a subclass of `ORKQuestionStep`. This class highlights the fact that the classes involved in obtaining informed consent are ResearchKit tasks and steps. As such, the application developer has the freedom to add custom ResearchKit tasks to the consent process for their application.

Similar to the visual consent and consent review step, consent sharing is implemented by including it in a task and then presenting that task with a task view controller, as follows:

```
// 1
let document = consentDocument()
// 2
let sharingConsentStep = ORKConsentSharingStep(identifier:
"ConsentSharingStep",
        investigatorShortDescription: "Institution",
        investigatorLongDescription: "Institution and its partners",
        localizedLearnMoreHTMLContent: "Learn more content")
let task = ORKOrderedTask(identifier: "ConsentTask", steps:
[sharingConsentStep])
let taskViewController = ORKTaskViewController(task: task,
taskRunUUID: nil)
taskViewController.delegate = self
presentViewController(taskViewController, animated: true, completion:
nil)
```

Consent process

So far, we have explored the steps of the consent process as individual ResearchKit tasks. Outside of the learning environment, the steps on the consent process will constitute one ResearchKit task. Assuming the earlier definition of the consent steps, they may be presented as one ResearchKit task, as follows:

```
let steps = [visualConsentStep, sharingConsentStep, reviewConsentStep]
let task = ORKOrderedTask(identifier: "ConsentTask", steps: steps)
let taskViewController = ORKTaskViewController(task: task,
taskRunUUID: nil)
taskViewController.delegate = self
presentViewController(taskViewController, animated: true, completion:
nil)
```

Obtaining results

The visual consent review, consent review, and data-sharing steps are ResearchKit steps that execute under a ResearchKit task. As such, these steps produce the result objects that the application may use as required. In setting up the task view controller, application specific a delegate for the view controller, as follows:

```
let task = ORKOrderedTask(identifier: "ConsentTask", steps:
[sharingConsentStep])
let taskViewController = ORKTaskViewController(task: task,
taskRunUUID: nil)
taskViewController.delegate = self
presentViewController(taskViewController, animated: true, completion:
nil)
```

The delegate for the task view controller must comply with the ORKTaskViewControllerDelegate protocol; the view controller defines a taskViewController:didFinishWithReasonerror: method that is invoked when the task has results. For consent, the following method definition extracts the results for each individual step:

```
func taskViewController(taskViewController: ORKTaskViewController,
didFinishWithReason reason: ORKTaskViewControllerFinishReason,
error: NSError?)
{
// 1
guard reason == .Completed else { return }
guard let taskResult = taskViewController.result else { return }
// 2
print("Task Id: ", taskResult.identifier)
```

```
if let consentSharingStepResult = taskResult.stepResultForStepIdentifi
er("ConsentSharingStep"),
    let sharingResult = consentSharingStepResult.firstResult as?
ORKChoiceQuestionResult
{
assert(sharingResult.questionType == .SingleChoice)
print("id", sharingResult.identifier)
print("Answer", sharingResult.choiceAnswers![0])
}


// 3
let visualConsentStepResult = taskResult.stepResultForStepIdentifier("
VisualConsentStep")
let visualResult = visualConsentStepResult?.firstResult //  No results
therefore will always be nil
    assert(visualResult == nil)


// 4
if let consentReviewStepResult = taskResult.stepResultForStepIdentifie
r("ConsentReviewStep"),
let reviewResult = consentReviewStepResult.firstResult as?
ORKConsentSignatureResult
{
print("Consented? ", reviewResult.consented)
if let signature = reviewResult.signature
{
print("Identifier:", signature.identifier)
print("Title: ", signature.title)
print("Given name: ", signature.givenName)
print("Family name: ", signature.familyName)
print("Signature image: ", signature.signatureImage)
print("Signature date: ", signature.signatureDate)
}
}
}
```

The explanation for the preceding code is as follows:

1. This method will be called when the task is completed, for any reason. For this example, we're only interested in successful completion and the task view controller must have a result object.

2. In order to obtain the results for the consent-sharing step, search for the step result using the `stepResultForStepIdentifier` method on the task result. This returns an `ORKStepResult`, whose dynamic type is `ORKChoiceQuestionResult`, a subclass of `ORKStepResult`. The `ORKChoiceQuestionResult` supports single-choice and multiple-choice questions. The data-sharing question is defined to accept a single-choice answer, therefore, the `choiceAnswers` array on the result object contains the participant's data-sharing preference.

The visual consent step produces a result object; however, it does not contain any actual results. This can be confirmed by taking a look at the step results for the `VisualConsentStep` step identifier and asserting the first result is `nil`.

1. The consent-review step produces a signature result object, an instance of `ORKConsentSignatureResult`. With this result object, the application can retrieve the participant's title, given name, family name, signature image, and the date on which the signing took place.

Summary

In this chapter, you learned how to obtain informed consent from the study participant by customizing ResearchKit's consent document.

In the next chapter, let's take a look at creating active tasks in depth.

5
Active Tasks

The primary role of ResearchKit is to engage the study participant in activities designed to elicit data in order to address questions posed by the study. Through the use of directed activities, ResearchKit-based applications may record data from device sensors as well as information directly entered by the user. ResearchKit is shipped with five built-in active tasks that serve as example tasks and may be used in an application.

The five active tasks included in ResearchKit are as follows:

- **Short walk task**: This task measures motor activities by recording device motion and pedometer data while the study participant takes a short walk
- **Two-finger tapping interval task**: This task measures motor activities by recording data from the multitouch display while the study participant is rapidly and alternatively tapping two targets on the device screen rapidly and alternatively
- **Fitness task**: This task measures fitness levels by recording device motion, location, heart rate, and data from the pedometer while the study participant is engaging in a multiphase walk
- **Spatial memory task**: This task measures cognitive ability by recording touch activities on the multitouch display while the study participant is engaged in a spatial-oriented game
- **Sustained phonation task**: This task records the study participant's voice while they are making a sustained sound

The sensors available to record data are as follows:

- Accelerometer
- Gyroscope
- Device motion
- Pedometer
- Multitouch display
- Location
- Heart rate via HealthKit

The five initial ResearchKit-based applications provide you with a wide range of activities, including the use of a few of these five active tasks:

Task	Application
Short walk task	mPower
Two-finger tapping task	mPower
Fitness task	MyHeart Counts
Spatial memory task	mPower
Sustained phonation task	mPower

Active tasks

Abstractly, the built-in active tasks consist of an instruction step (ORKInstructionStep), a *get ready* countdown step (ORKCountdownStep), task-specific step or steps, followed by a conclusion step (ORKCompletionStep). These tasks are instantiated following the same generic creation pattern employed by ResearchKit:

```
// 1
let task = ORKOrderedTask.fitnessCheckTaskWithIdentifier
("FitnessTask",
         intendedUseDescription: "Blah, blah",
         walkDuration: 30.0,
         restDuration: 15.0,
         options: .None)
// 2
let taskViewController = ORKTaskViewController(task: task,
taskRunUUID: nil)
// 3
taskViewController.delegate = self
// 4
let defaultFileManager = NSFileManager.defaultManager()
```

```
let documentDirectoryURL = defaultFileManager.URLsForDirectory
(.DocumentDirectory,
                          inDomains: .UserDomainMask)
taskViewController.outputDirectory = documentDirectoryURL.first!
// 5
presentViewController(taskViewController, animated: true, completion:
nil)
```

The explanation of the above code is given below:

1. Instantiate the task. Class methods on ORKOrderedTask are used to instantiate the built-in active tasks.

2. Instantiate the view controller with the instantiated task.

3. Set the task view controller's delegate property. This is required in order to process collected data at the conclusion of the task.

4. Assign parameters to the task view controller such as the delegate. In this particular case, we are setting the output directory that tells the view controller where to write the data recorded from the task.

5. Present the view controller.

At the conclusion of a task, each step will have a result object even if the step did not produce result data. For steps that produce a result, the resulting object will be an object whose type is a subclass of ORKResult. For the built-in active tasks, the step results will be one of the following:

- ORKFileResult: This references a file produced during a task.

- ORKSpatialSpanMemoryResult: This records the result of a spatial span memory step. This includes the score displayed to the user, number of rounds, number of failures, and an array of result records.

- ORKTappingIntervalResult: This records the results of a tapping-interval task. These results include an array of touch samples (timestamp, location, and target identifier) and the geometry of the task.

The task view controller maintains the results for each step of the task. The delegate for the task view controller will be given the opportunity to process data at the conclusion of a task. The delegate must comply with ORKTaskViewControllerDelegate and implement the taskViewController:didFinishWithReason:error method. This method will be invoked at the conclusion of the task and, in most cases, it should dismiss the view controller. A generic form of this method is as follows:

```
func taskViewController(taskViewController: ORKTaskViewController,
        didFinishWithReason reason: ORKTaskViewControllerFinishReason,
        error: NSError?)
```

```
{
    let taskResult = taskViewController.result

    // Process first results
    let stepResult = taskResult.stepResultForStepIdentifier(<step
identifier>)

    if let result = stepResult?.firstResult as? <result type, such as
ORKFileResult>
    {
        <process result>
    }

    // Process second results, if any
    ...
    dismissViewControllerAnimated(true, completion: nil)
}
```

The task view controller will invoke the `taskViewController:`
`didFinishWithReason:error` method on the delegate when an unrecoverable error
occurs or when the user has cancelled the task. Similar to the successful completion
of the task, the delegate should dismiss the view controller.

The `taskViewController:recorder:didFailWithError` method on the delegate
will be called whenever the recorder detects an error. This will occur when sensor
data is not available or there is insufficient disk space to record the results.

Short walk task

The short walk task asks the study participant to take a short walk, which is split
into two legs with an optional resting phase. The presentation of this task uses the
pedometer's step count as a countdown indicator. When the participant has taken the
specified number of steps, they are asked to turn around and return to their starting
point. When the second leg of the walk is completed, the participant is asked to stand
still for a given period of time in order to collect baseline data.

The short walk task has two options specific to the task:

- **Number of steps**: This is the number of steps that the participant should take
  for each leg of the walk
- **Rest duration**: This is the number of seconds that the participant is asked to
  stand still in order to collect baseline data.

The `options` parameter to the task allows you to exclude the following:

Options	Enumeration
Exclude the instruction step	`ORKPredefinedTaskOptionExcludeInstructions`
Exclude the conclusion step	`ORKPredefinedTaskOptionExcludeConclusion`
Exclude the recording of pedometer data	`ORKPredefinedTaskOptionExcludePedometer`
Exclude the recording of accelerometer data	`ORKPredefinedTaskOptionExcludeAccelerometer`
Exclude the recording of device motion data	`ORKPredefinedTaskOptionExcludeDeviceMotion`

Sample code

Here is an example of a short walk task with 20 steps per leg followed by a 60-second rest interval:

```
let task = ORKOrderedTask.shortWalkTaskWithIdentifier("ShortWalkTask",
        intendedUseDescription: "Blah, blah",
        numberOfStepsPerLeg: 20,
        restDuration: 60.0,
        options: .None)
let taskViewController = ORKTaskViewController(task: task,
taskRunUUID: nil)
taskViewController.delegate = self
let defaultFileManager = NSFileManager.defaultManager()
let documentDirectoryURL = defaultFileManager.URLsForDirectory
(.DocumentDirectory,
                        inDomains: .UserDomainMask)
taskViewController.outputDirectory = documentDirectoryURL.first!
presentViewController(taskViewController, animated: true, completion:
nil)
```

Results

The short walk task may record data from the accelerometer, gyroscope, and device motion. The following code snippet is a generic way of processing the results of this task:

```
func taskViewController(taskViewController: ORKTaskViewController,
        didFinishWithReason reason: ORKTaskViewControllerFinishReason,
        error: NSError?)
{
    let taskResult = taskViewController.result

    // Process first results
```

```
    let outboundStepResult = taskResult.stepResultForStepIdentifier
(ORKShortWalkOutboundStepIdentifier)

    if let result = outboundStepResult?.firstResult as? ORKFileResult
    {
        <process result>
    }
    //  Process second results
    let returnStepResult = taskResult.stepResultForStepIdentifier
(ORKShortWalkReturnStepIdentifier)
    if let result = returnStepResult?.firstResult as? ORKFileResult
    {
        <process result>
    }
    //  Process third results
    let restStepResult = taskResult.stepResultForStepIdentifier
(ORKShortWalkRestStepIdentifier)
    if let result = restStepResult?.firstResult as? ORKFileResult
    {
        <process result>
    }
    dismissViewControllerAnimated(true, completion: nil)
}
```

Screenshot

The following figure shows you the screenshots of the short walk task:

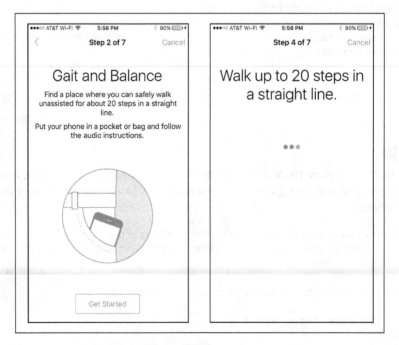

Two-finger tapping interval task

The two-finger tapping task presents two circular targets on the device screen. The participant is asked to tap the targets rapidly and alternatively with two fingers on the same hand. Once the task begins, a progress indicator is displayed along with a tap count.

The two-finger tapping task has one specific task parameter that an application can set: the duration. This parameter specifies in seconds how long the active step of this task runs while data is collected.

The options parameter to the task allows you to exclude the following:

Options	Enumeration
Exclude the instruction step	ORKPredefinedTaskOptionExcludeInstructions
Exclude the conclusion step	ORKPredefinedTaskOptionExcludeConclusion
Exclude the recording of accelerometer data	ORKPredefinedTaskOptionExcludeAccelerometer

Sample code

Here is an example of the two-finger tapping task that exercises the active phase of the task for 60 seconds:

```
let task = ORKOrderedTask.twoFingerTappingIntervalTaskWithIdentifier(
"TappingTask",
            intendedUseDescription: "Blah, blah",
            duration: 60.0,
            options: .None)
let taskViewController = ORKTaskViewController(task: task,
taskRunUUID: nil)
taskViewController.delegate = self
let defaultFileManager = NSFileManager.defaultManager()
let documentDirectoryURL = defaultFileManager.URLsForDirectory
(.DocumentDirectory,
                            inDomains: .UserDomainMask)
taskViewController.outputDirectory = documentDirectoryURL.first!
presentViewController(taskViewController, animated: true, completion:
nil)
```

Results

The two-finger tapping task may record data from the accelerometer and multitouch display. The following code snippet is a generic way of processing the results of this task:

```
func taskViewController(taskViewController: ORKTaskViewController,
        didFinishWithReason reason: ORKTaskViewControllerFinishReason,
        error: NSError?)
{
    let taskResult = taskViewController.result

    // Process first results
    let stepResult = taskResult.stepResultForStepIdentifier
(ORKTappingStepIdentifier)

    if let result = stepResult?.firstResult as? ORKFileResult
    {
        <process result>
    }

    dismissViewControllerAnimated(true, completion: nil)
}
```

Screenshot

The following figure shows you the screenshots of the two-finger tapping interval task:

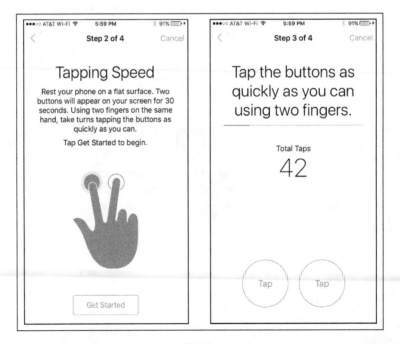

Fitness task

The fitness task asks the participant to walk for a specified walk duration and, if a heart-rate monitor is detected, asks the participant to sit still for a specified rest duration. During the walk phase, the task will present the accumulated distance as a progress indicator and the participant's heart rate.

The first time that the participant attempts the fitness task, they will be asked to grant permission to collect certain types of data between the instruction and countdown steps. HealthKit will present its permission view in order to obtain permission to record heart-rate data. Then, the participant will be given the opportunity to grant permission for the application to access Motion & Fitness Activity.

The fitness task has two options specific to the task:

1. Walk duration: This is the duration of the walk phase of the task in seconds. If the walk duration is equal to zero, this step is not included in the task.

2. Rest duration: This is the duration of the rest phase of the task in seconds. If the rest duration is equal to zero, this step is not included in the task.

The options parameter to the task allows you to exclude the following:

Options	Enumeration
Exclude the instruction step	ORKPredefinedTaskOptionExcludeInstructions
Exclude the conclusion step	ORKPredefinedTaskOptionExcludeConclusion
Exclude the recording of pedometer data	ORKPredefinedTaskOptionExcludePedometer
Exclude the recording of accelerometer data	ORKPredefinedTaskOptionExcludeAccelerometer
Exclude the recording of device motion data	ORKPredefinedTaskOptionExcludeDeviceMotion
Exclude the recording of location data	ORKPredefinedTaskOptionExcludeLocation

Note: Location data may be considered protected health information and processing of the data may be required prior to uploading the data to a data-collection service.

Sample code

Here is an example of the fitness task with a two-minute walk phase and 30-second rest phase:

```
let task = ORKOrderedTask.fitnessCheckTaskWithIdentifier
("FitnessTask",
                    intendedUseDescription: "Blah, blah",
                    walkDuration: 120.0,
                    restDuration: 30.0,
                    options: .None)
let taskViewController = ORKTaskViewController(task: task,
taskRunUUID: nil)
taskViewController.delegate = self
let defaultFileManager = NSFileManager.defaultManager()
let documentDirectoryURL = defaultFileManager.URLsForDirectory
(.DocumentDirectory,
                        inDomains: .UserDomainMask)
taskViewController.outputDirectory = documentDirectoryURL.first!
presentViewController(taskViewController, animated: true, completion:
nil)
```

Results

The fitness task may record data from the accelerometer, device motion, pedometer, location, and heart rate. The following code snippet is a generic way of processing the results of this task:

```
func taskViewController(taskViewController: ORKTaskViewController,
        didFinishWithReason reason: ORKTaskViewControllerFinishReason,
        error: NSError?)
{
    let taskResult = taskViewController.result
    // Process first results
    let stepResult = taskResult.stepResultForStepIdentifier
(ORKFitnessWalkStepIdentifier)
    if let result = stepResult?.firstResult as? ORKFileResult
    {
        <process result>
    }
    // Process the second results
    let stepResult = taskResult.stepResultForStepIdentifier
(ORKFitnessRestStepIdentifier)
    if let result = stepResult?.firstResult as? ORKFileResult
    {
        <process results>
    }
    dismissViewControllerAnimated(true, completion: nil)
}
```

Screenshot

The following figure shows you the screenshots of the fitness task:

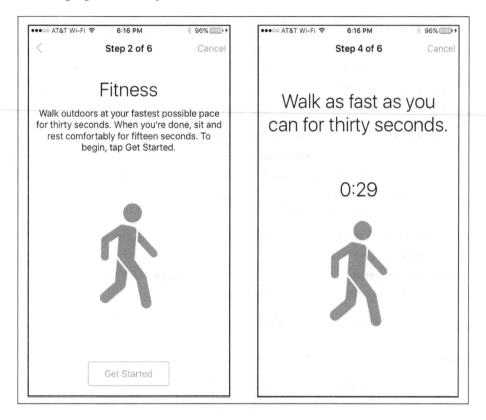

Spatial memory task

The spatial memory task is a game-like active task that may be used to assess visuospatial skills. This task asks the participant to repeat sequences of patterns that increase in length for each subsequent round of the task. Using a demonstration phase, the task presents a grid of images and highlights a number of the images in a sequence. The participant is then asked to tap the images in the same sequence as the demonstration phase. If the participant taps the correct sequence of images, the length of the pattern sequence increases for the next round. If the participant makes a mistake, the length of the pattern sequence decreases for the next round. The rounds continue until either the maximum number of rounds have been played or the maximum number of failures have been reached.

The spatial memory task has a number of options specific to this task:

1. **Initial span**: This is the length of the initial sequence of patterns for the first round.

2. **Minimum span**: This is the minimum length of a sequence of patterns. The options come into play when the participant repeats the presented sequence of the pattern incorrectly.

3. **Maximum span**: This is the maximum length of a sequence of patterns.

4. **Play speed**: This will control the speed of play.

5. **Maximum tests**: This is the maximum number of rounds.

6. **Maximum consecutive failures**: This is the maximum number of consecutive failures that the participant may make before the task is terminated.

7. **Custom target image**: This is the image to use within the grid of patterns. By default, the image is a flower.

8. **Custom target plural name**: This is the display name associated with the custom target image.

9. **Require reversal**: This is an indicator as to whether the participant is required to tap the sequence in reverse order.

The `options` parameter to the task allows you to exclude the following:

Options	Enumeration
Exclude the instruction step	`ORKPredefinedTaskOptionExcludeInstructions`
Exclude the conclusion step	`ORKPredefinedTaskOptionExcludeConclusion`

Sample Code

```
let task = ORKOrderedTask.spatialSpanMemoryTaskWithIdentifier
("SpatialMemoryTask",
                    intendedUseDescription: "Blah, blah",
                    initialSpan: 2,
                    minimumSpan: 1,
                    maximumSpan: 4,
                    playSpeed: 0.5,
                    maxTests: 6,
                    maxConsecutiveFailures: 4,
                    customTargetImage: nil,
                    customTargetPluralName: nil,
                    requireReversal: true,
                    options: .None)
```

```
let taskViewController = ORKTaskViewController(task: task,
taskRunUUID: nil)
taskViewController.delegate = self
let defaultFileManager = NSFileManager.defaultManager()
let documentDirectoryURL = defaultFileManager.URLsForDirectory
(.DocumentDirectory,
                                inDomains: .UserDomainMask)
taskViewController.outputDirectory = documentDirectoryURL.first!
presentViewController(taskViewController, animated: true, completion:
nil)
```

Results

The spatial memory task may record data from the multitouch display. The
following code snippet is a generic way of processing the results of this task:

```
func taskViewController(taskViewController: ORKTaskViewController,
        didFinishWithReason reason: ORKTaskViewControllerFinishReason,
        error: NSError?)
{
    let taskResult = taskViewController.result
    // Process first results
    let stepResult = taskResult.stepResultForStepIdentifier(ORKSpatial
SpanMemoryStepIdentifier)
    if let result = stepResult?.firstResult as?
ORKSpatialSpanMemoryResult
    {
        <process result>
    }

    dismissViewControllerAnimated(true, completion: nil)
}
```

Screenshot

The following figure shows you the screenshots of the spatial memory task:

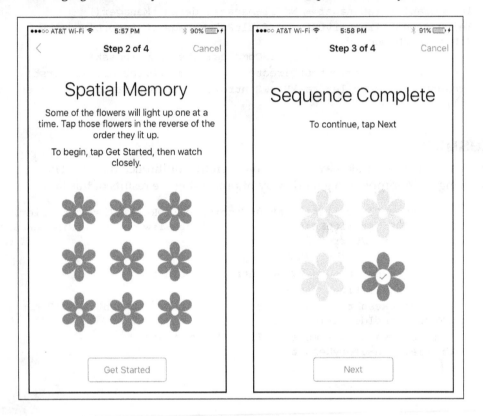

Sustained phonation task

The sustained phonation task asks the participant to make a sound with their voice while the task records sounds via the microphone. During the presentation of the task, a wave form is displayed providing an indication of sound levels.

The first time that the participant performs the task, they will be asked to grant permission to access the microphone. This will occur between the instruction and countdown steps.

The sustained phonation task has four options specific to the task:

1. Speech instruction: This describes what the participant needs to do when the recording begins.

2. Short speech instruction: This is the instructional content displayed during the recording phase of the task.

3. Duration: This is the length of time for the recording phase in seconds.

4. Recording settings: This is a dictionary of settings to control the recording of the participant's voice. See AV Foundation Audio Settings Constants for possible values.

The `options` parameter to the task allows you to exclude the following:

Options	Enumeration
Exclude the instruction step	`ORKPredefinedTaskOptionExcludeInstructions`
Exclude the conclusion step	`ORKPredefinedTaskOptionExcludeConclusion`

Sample code

Here is an example of the sustained phonation task asking the participant to say `Ahhh` for 15 seconds:

```
let task = ORKOrderedTask.audioTaskWithIdentifier("SustainedPhonation
Task",
                    intendedUseDescription: "Blah, blah",
                    speechInstruction: "Please say \"Ahhh\" for 15
seconds",
                    shortSpeechInstruction: "Please say \"Ahhh\"",
                    duration: 15.0,
                    recordingSettings: nil,
                    options: .None)
let taskViewController = ORKTaskViewController(task: task,
taskRunUUID: nil)
taskViewController.delegate = self
let defaultFileManager = NSFileManager.defaultManager()
let documentDirectoryURL = defaultFileManager.URLsForDirectory
(.DocumentDirectory,
                          inDomains: .UserDomainMask)
taskViewController.outputDirectory = documentDirectoryURL.first!
presentViewController(taskViewController, animated: true, completion:
nil)
```

Results

The sustained phonation task records data from the microphone. The following code snippet is a generic way of processing the results of this task:

```
func taskViewController(taskViewController: ORKTaskViewController,
        didFinishWithReason reason: ORKTaskViewControllerFinishReason,
        error: NSError?)
{
    guard reason == .Completed else { return }
```

```
    let taskResult       = taskViewController.result
    let audioStepResult = taskResult.stepResultForStepIdentifier
("audio")
    if let audioResult = audioStepResult?.firstResult as?
ORKFileResult
    {
        print("Content type ", audioResult.contentType)
        print("URL: ", audioResult.fileURL)
    }
    dismissViewControllerAnimated(true, completion: nil)
}
```

Screenshot

The following figure shows you the screenshots of the sustained phonation task:

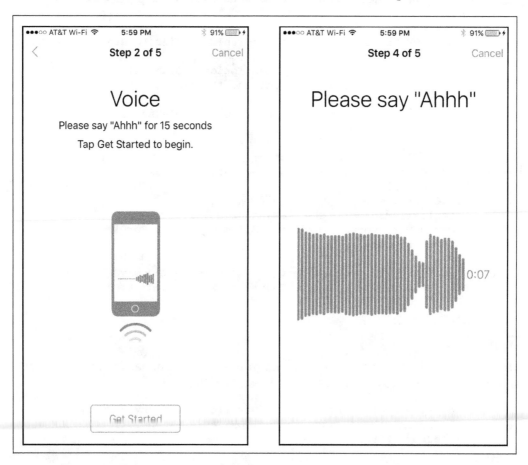

Data formats

A number of the built-in active tasks record data to files. With the exception of audio data, the data stored in these files are written in the JSON format. These data categories are as follows:

- Pedometer
- Location
- Device motion
- Accelerometer
- Audio data

Pedometer data

The collected pedometer data will be an array of tuples consisting of the following:

1. **Start date**: This is the initial date and time over which this dataset was collected.
2. **End date**: This is the end date and time over which this dataset was collected.
3. **Number of steps**: This is the step count that the participant took for this dataset.
4. **Distance**: This is the distance that the participant traveled for this dataset.
5. **Floors ascended**: This is the number of floors that the participant ascended for this dataset.
6. **Floors descended**: This is the number of floors that the participant descended for this dataset.

 Note: Pedometer data is recorded in discrete chunks over a period of time and not as a stream of data. A single instance of pedometer data represents participant behavior between a start and end date and time.

The following is an example of pedometer data:

```
{
    "items":
    [
        {
            "floorsAscended":0,
            "floorsDescended":0,
            "endDate":"2015-10-11T06:18:39-0700",
            "startDate":"2015-10-11T06:18:30-0700",
            "numberOfSteps":8,
            "distance":10.46454413188621
```

```
        },
        {
            . . .
        }
    ]
}
```

Location data

The collected location data will be an array of timestamped tuples of the following:

1. **Timestamp**: This is the time at which the location was determined
2. **Coordinate**: This consists of latitude, longitude, and horizontal accuracy
3. **Altitude**: This is measured in meters
4. **Vertical accuracy**: This is the accuracy of the altitude measured in meters
5. **Course**: This is the compass direction measured in degrees
6. **Speed**: This is the instantaneous speed measured in meters per second
7. **Floor**: This is the logical floor of the building

Device motion data

The collected device motion data will be an array of timestamped tuples of the following:

1. Attitude consisting of x, y, z, and w values
2. Rotation rate consisting of x, y, and z values
3. Gravity consisting of x, y, and z values
4. User acceleration consisting of x, y, and z values
5. Magnetic field consisting of x, y, z, and accuracy values

The following is an example of device motion data:

```
{
    "items":
    [
        {
            "attitude":
            {
                "y":0.1859032222233062912,
                "w":0.9462335956470929408,
                "z":-0.0022928578837123904,
                "x":0.2647200733576715264
```

```
        },
        "timestamp":129887.48952879169536,
        "rotationRate":
        {
            "x":0.3697428107261658112,
            "y":-0.79918390512466432,
            "z":-0.6724496483802796032
        },
        "userAcceleration":
        {
            "x":0.01360850408673286144,
            "y":-0.016830960288643837952,
            "z":-0.02654945105314254336
        },
        "gravity":
        {
            "x":0.35302966833114624,
            "y":-0.50012153387069696,
            "z":-0.7907265424728393728
        },
        "magneticField":
        {
            "y":0,
            "z":0,
            "x":0,
            "accuracy":-1
        }
    },
    {
        ...
    }
    ]
}
```

Accelerometer data

The collected accelerometer data will be an array of timestamped three-axis acceleration values (x, y, and z).

The following is an example of accelerometer data:

```
{
"items":
    [
        {
```

```
            "y":-0.722808837890625024,
            "timestamp":129795.28485074997248,
            "z":-0.7686004638671874048,
            "x":-0.07594299316406249472
        },
        {

            "y":-0.718643188476562432,
            "timestamp":129795.2946787500032,
            "z":-0.7648620605468750848,
            "x":-0.0732574462890625024
        },
        {

            . . .

        }
    ]
}
```

Audio data

For tasks that use ORKAudioStep (for example, the sustained phonation task), ORKAudioRecorder is configured with the following default settings:

1. The MPEG-4 AAC format
2. Minimum audio quality for sample rate conversion
3. Two channels
4. 44100.0 hertz sample rate

The recorded audio file will be found on the disk at the conclusion of the task.

Summary

The built-in active tasks provided by ResearchKit provide you with an excellent vehicle to learn about ResearchKit and its architecture, and the implementation of a variety of tasks that employ a multitude of sensors.

6
Navigable and Custom Tasks

In the previous chapters, we looked at the various basic building blocks of ResearchKit applications such as ordered tasks, consent, active tasks, and so on. In this chapter, we will be studying the advanced areas of ResearchKit.

Specifically, in this chapter, you will learn how to create navigable tasks and custom tasks.

Navigable ordered tasks

In *Chapter 3, Building Surveys*, we looked at creating simple surveys using `ORKOrderedTask`. This method is sufficient to convert most of the paper surveys to a ResearchKit app. However, the advantage of presenting a clinical survey on the phone is that we can adapt the survey based on the responses for the previous questions. For example, in a smoking habits survey, when the user answers that they does not smoke, the survey can choose not to ask how many cigarettes do they smoke per day. The `ORKNavigableOrderedTask` allows you to adapt the questions based on the answers the user chooses.

The `ORKNavigableOrderedTask` is a subclass of `ORKOrderedTask` and it adds conditional step navigation to the ordered tasks. We can add conditional steps in `ORKNavigableOrderedTask` by attaching the navigation rules to the specific steps. There are two types of navigation rules, as follows:

- Navigation rules with predicates are represented by the `ORKPredicateStepNavigationRule` class. They allow us to navigate to different steps in a survey based on the result predicates represented by `ORKResultPredicate`.

- Direct navigation rules (represented by `ORKDirectStepNavigationRule`) allow us to directly jump to different steps in a survey without any conditions.

In order to learn navigable ordered tasks, let's look at a reduced version of the survey that we presented in *Chapter 3, Building Surveys,* to illustrate the use of the navigable tasks. Open the `NavigableTask.swift` file to follow along:

```swift
func showNavigableTask()
{
    //1 - Declare Constants for step identifiers
    let instructionID = "Instruction Step"
    let question1ID = "question 1"
    let question2ID = "question 2"
    let completionChoice1ID = "completionChoice 1"
    let completionChoice2ID = "completionChoice 2"

    //2 - Set up steps array
    let instStep = ORKInstructionStep(identifier: instructionID)
    instStep.title = "Navigable Survey"
    instStep.detailText = "This survey demonstrates
ORKNavigableOrderedTask"

    let question1 = ORKQuestionStep(identifier: question1ID,
title: "Have you ever been diagnosed w Softwareitis?", answer:
ORKAnswerFormat.booleanAnswerFormat())

    let question2 = ORKQuestionStep(identifier: question2ID, title:
"How many apps do you download pweek?", answer: ORKAnswerFormat.
integerAnswerFormatWithUnit("Apps per week"))

    let completionStep1 = ORKCompletionStep(identifier:
completionChoice1ID)
    completionStep1.title = "Thank you for letting us know that you
are Softwareitis free!"

    let completionStep2 = ORKCompletionStep(identifier:
completionChoice2ID)
    completionStep2.title = "Thank you for taking our survey!"

    //3 - Instantiate ORKNavigableOrderedTask
    let task = ORKNavigableOrderedTask(identifier: "first
survey", steps: [instStep, question1, qtion2, completionStep1,
completionStep2])
```

```
//4 - show task view controller
    let taskViewController = ORKTaskViewController(task: task,
taskRunUUID: nil)
    taskViewController.delegate = self
    presentViewController(taskViewController, animated: true,
completion: nil)
  }
```

In the preceding `showNavigableTask` method, we create an ordered task with five steps: one instruction step:

- Question step 1: This asks the user if they have Softwareitis
- Question step 2: This asks the user the number of apps that they download per week
- Completion step 1: For users who answered that they don't have Softwareitis
- Completion step 2: For users who answered that they do have the Softwareitis condition.

Ideally Question step 2 should be presented only when the user says that they have Softwareitis condition, as follows:

1. Declares constants for step identifiers so that they can be reused in navigation rules.
2. Creates array of five steps.
3. Creates the `ORKNavigableOrderedTask` task object with steps created earlier.
4. Presents the task view controller with the created task.

So far, this code is identical to creating a survey with `ORKOrderedTask`. If we build and run, we will see that `ORKNavigableTask` behaves exactly same way as `ORKOrderedTask`-all the questions are presented one after the other without any conditional jumps.

Now, let's add our first navigation rule using the following code. Insert the below between steps 3 and 4 above:

```
//1
let question1Predicate = ORKResultPredicate.
predicateForBooleanQuestionResultWithResultSelector(ORKResultSelector
(resultIdentifier: question1ID), expectedAnswer: false)

//2
```

```
let predicatedNavigationRule = ORKPredicateStepNavigationRule
(resultPredicates: [question1Predicate], destinationStepIdentifiers:
[completionChoice1ID])

//3
task.setNavigationRule(predicatedNavigationRule,
forTriggerStepIdentifier: question1ID)
```

The preceding lines of code adds conditional rule to skip question 2 if the user has answered that they don't have Softwareitis in the first question:

1. Creates an ORKResultPredicate object with a predicate that checks whether the result of question step 1 is false. Refer to the ORKResultPredicate documentation to learn about the different predicate types. The ORKResultSelector object helps ORKResultPredicate locate the result in ORKStepResult using the step identifier in the resultIdentifier parameter. Note that most of the times, you would be using the ORKResultSelector(resultIdentifier:) method to locate the result for a particular step, where resultIdentifier is same as the identifier of the step. In case, a form (with multiple questions) is used for a step, the ORKResultSelector(stepIdentifier:resultIdentifier:) method should be used to locate the appropriate answer for the predicate.

2. Creates an ORKPredicateStepNavigationRule object with the predicate and the identifier of the desired destination step if the predicate is met (in this case, we want to jump to *completion step 1*). Please note that the method takes an array of predicates and destination identifiers. Therefore, you can create a navigation rule with multiple predicates and destination identifiers for a single step.

3. Adds the navigation rule created in 2 to question step 1 by providing question1ID in the trigger step identifier.

If we build and run the preceding code, we can see that a conditional step is added in *question step 1*. However, we still have the following two problems:

1. When the user chooses that they don't have Softwareitis, question step 2 is skipped and jumped to completion step 1. However, after completion step 1, we still show completion step 2. Ideally, the survey should complete without showing completion step 2.

2. When the user chooses that they do have Softwareitis, completion step 1 is presented after question step 2. Ideally, completion step 1 should be skipped for this user. Let's fix all of these problems using the `ORKDirectStepNavigationRule` objects, as follows:

```
//1
let directNavigationRule1 = ORKDirectStepNavigationRule
(destinationStepIdentifier: completionChoice2ID)
task.setNavigationRule(directNavigationRule1,
forTriggerStepIdentifier: question2ID)

//2
let directNavigationRule2 = ORKDirectStepNavigationRule
(destinationStepIdentifier: ORKNullStepIdentifier)
task.setNavigationRule(directNavigationRule2,
forTriggerStepIdentifier: completionChoice1ID)
```

The following is the explanation of the preceding code:

1. Creates a direct navigation rule that skips completion step 1 after question step 2. It sets the destination step identifier as `completionChoice2ID` and trigger step identifier as `question2ID`.

2. Creates a direct navigation rule that skips completion step 2 and takes the user to the end of the survey after completion step 1. The `ORKNullStepIdentifier` is a predefined constant in ResearchKit to indicate the end of task.

With the above code, the navigable ordered task is fully complete and functional.

The results from the navigable ordered tasks are similar to ordered tasks; however, they will contain results from only the steps that were presented to the user.

Custom tasks

While navigable ordered tasks offer flexibility to skip steps, this may not be enough for more complex tasks. In such cases, ResearchKit allows you to build the custom tasks. Custom tasks can be built by creating objects that conform to the `ORKTask` protocol. These tasks provide the ultimate flexibility in dynamically choosing the next step based on the results from the previous steps. In the initial five ResearchKit apps that Apple announced, custom tasks were used to generate dynamic surveys based on the data received from the backend server and the answers provided by the users.

The ORKTask protocol has one non-optional property and two non-optional methods that need to be implemented in order to conform to this protocol. The ORKTaskViewController calls these methods on the custom task object to obtain relevant steps and dynamically present step view controllers to accomplish the step, as follows:

```
//1
public var identifier: String

//2
public func stepAfterStep(step: ORKStep?, withResult result:
ORKTaskResult) -> ORKStep?

//3
 public func stepBeforeStep(step: ORKStep?, withResult result:
ORKTaskResult) -> ORKStep?
```

1. This identifier is same as the identifiers that we have been using so far to identify any specific task.

2. This method needs to return the next step based on the current step provided in the step parameter. The results of the earlier steps are available in the result parameter. Using both step and result parameters, the custom task object can dynamically choose the next step to be presented to the user.

3. This method needs to return the previous step based on the step and result parameters. This method can always return nil if you do not want to support going back to the previous steps. Note that supporting going back in custom tasks could add significant complexity to the design of custom tasks as the users could potentially take different series of steps than the one that they have already taken after going back. The design of custom task needs to accommodate these cases.

Caution: Custom tasks support looping back to the previous steps. In such tasks, there is a potential for infinite loop back and the tasks might not end. Also, such tasks could be confusing for the users. ResearchKit documentation recommends using ORKOrderedTask or ORKNavigableOrderedTask for most of the tasks and avoid using custom tasks, if possible.

In order to learn custom tasks, let's take look at a fictitious survey with 11 questions. The first question presents the user with choice whether they want to see all the remaining 10 questions, odd numbered questions, or even numbered questions. Depending on the answer to the first question, the user is presented with all, odd, or even questions. You can find the `Softwareitis.xcodeproj` project corresponding to this chapter in the `Chapter\_6/Softwareitis` folder of the RKBook. Open the `CustomTask.swift` and `EvenOddTask.swift` files to follow along.

The `EvenOddTask` is the object that conforms to the `ORKTask` protocol and a subclass of `NSObject`. The following code shows the relevant portions of this class:

```
class EvenOddTask: NSObject, ORKTask
{
    //1 - Constants and Properties
    var identifier = "EvenOddTask"
    var stepsDictionary : [String : ORKStep] = [:] //Stores all the
steps necessary for this task
    let firstQuestionID = "first question"
    var questionsFilter = QuestionsFilter.all

    //2 - Initializer
    override init() {
        super.init()
        fillStepsDictionary()
    }

    func fillStepsDictionary()
    {
        //Generate first question step
        let textChoice1 = ORKTextChoice(text: "All", value: 1)
        let textChoice2 = ORKTextChoice(text: "Odd", value: 2)
        let textChoice3 = ORKTextChoice(text: "Even", value: 3)
        let answerFormat4 = ORKNumericAnswerFormat.choiceAnswerFormatW
ithStyle(ORKChoiceAnswerStyle.SingleChoice, textChoices: [textChoice1,
textChoice2, textChoice3])
        let firstQuestionStep = ORKQuestionStep(identifier:
firstQuestionID, title: "Which type of questions you want?", answer:
answerFormat4)
        firstQuestionStep.optional = false

        stepsDictionary[firstQuestionID] = firstQuestionStep
```

```
        //Generate 10 question steps
        for i in 1...10
        {
            let identifier = "Question \(i)"
            let question = ORKQuestionStep(identifier: identifier,
title: "This is \(identifier).", answer: ORKAnswerFormat.
booleanAnswerFormat())
            stepsDictionary[identifier] = question
        }
    }


    //3 - Step After Step Method
    func stepAfterStep(step: ORKStep?, withResult result:
ORKTaskResult) -> ORKStep? {
        if let stepValue = step
        {
            //Set up questionsFilter by accessing the result of first
question
            if let firstQuestionStepResult = result.
stepResultForStepIdentifier(firstQuestionID)?.
results?.first as? ORKChoiceQuestionResult,
answer = firstQuestionStepResult.
choiceAnswers?.first as? Int
            {
                switch answer
                {
                case 1:
                    questionsFilter = .all
                case 2:
                    questionsFilter = .odd
                case 3:
                    questionsFilter = .even
                default:
                    questionsFilter = .all
                }
            }

            //Calculate next identifier
            if let stepIdValue = stepIdentifierAfterIdentifier
(stepValue.identifier)
            {
                return stepsDictionary[stepIdValue]
            }
            else
            {
```

```
                return nil
            }
        }
        else
        {
            return stepsDictionary[firstQuestionID]
        }
    }

    //4 - Step before step method. Returns nil as we are not
supporting going back yet.
    func stepBeforeStep(step: ORKStep?, withResult result:
ORKTaskResult) -> ORKStep? {
        return nil
    }

    //Other helper methods are skipped. Please look at sample code.
    //....
}
```

The explanation for the preceding code is as follows:

1. Declares constants and properties. Please note that the `identifier` property is set as a constant `EvenOddTask`.

2. The initializer creates a steps dictionary to store all the potential steps that are necessary for this custom task.

3. Implements the `stepAfterStep` method. It evaluates the answer from question to set the `questionsFilter` property to all, or even, or odd. Then, it uses a helper `stepIdentifierAfterIdentifier` method to calculate the next step based on the `questionsFilter` property.

4. Implements the `stepBeforeStep` method. Currently it returns nil. This case does not support going back to the previous step.

Now that the custom task class is declared, it can be presented using a very few lines of code in `customTask.swift`, as shown in the following:

```
func showCustomTask()
{
    //1
    let customTask = EvenOddTask()

    //2
```

```
    let taskViewController = ORKTaskViewController(task: customTask,
taskRunUUID: nil)
    taskViewController.delegate = self
    presentViewController(taskViewController, animated: true,
completion: nil)
}
```

The explanation of the preceding code is as follows:

1. Instantiates an EvenOddTask object.

2. Presents the task using a new task view controller just like any other ordered tasks.

3. The EvenOddTask is already designed to support going back to the previous steps. Please uncomment the commented lines stepBeforeStep method and comment out the return nil line, you should be able to enable going back to the appropriate steps based on the questionsFilter property.

4. The ORKTask supports showing the progress of the current task using the ORKProgressTask struct and progressOfCurrentStep (step:, withResult result:) optional protocol methods. Refer to the documentation to learn how to use these methods to show the progress to the user.

Summary

In this chapter, you learned how to create navigable ordered tasks and custom tasks to create dynamic surveys that are customized to the users' responses.

In the next chapter, we will take a look at how to utilize the results produced from the tasks by sending them to backend server.

7

Backend Service

In the previous chapters, our main focus was on utilizing ResearchKit's classes such as ORKTask and ORKTaskViewController to make users accomplish various types of tasks: ordered, consent, active, navigable, and custom tasks. In this chapter, we will focus on utilizing the results generated in these tasks.

Why is backend service needed?

The main purpose of a ResearchKit-based clinical research app is to collect and analyze the results generated in various tasks performed by users. For example, an asthma-related clinical study app might require the users to respond to a weekly survey on their condition. The researchers can then analyze the survey responses to discover trends and patterns. In order to collect, manage, and analyze the data, a backend service or server is needed. The ResearchKit framework does not provide such a backend service. It is solely the responsibility of the application to provide backend support.

A backend service can provide the following basic services to a ResearchKit app:

- User account creation and management
- Data collection, management, and analysis
- The anonymization of the collected data so that it can be shared with a larger research community

On top of the preceding basic services, it can also provide the following advanced services:

- The segmentation of users based on their task results
- The customization of tasks and surveys
- The customization of the schedule of the tasks

ResearchKit's architecture allows us to connect to backend services that provide both basic and advanced services.

Security and privacy

A participant's privacy and data security must have the highest priority while designing in-house or choosing a third-party provider for the backend service. Moreover, such a service should be compliant with the local health data privacy laws (for example, *HIPAA* in the U.S.). Note that Apple strongly recommends not using iCloud for ResearchKit's backend service.

Introduction to Sage Bionetworks and the Bridge service

Sage Bionetworks, a non-profit biomedical research organization founded in 2009, has the mission to improve the understanding and treatment of human diseases through data-driven predictive modeling. In order to support this mission, Sage provided the cloud-based platform that served as the destination for data collected from the initial ResearchKit-based applications. This platform, called `Bridge`, facilitates the gathering of consistently structured data from the study participants and enables the aggregation, distribution, and reuse of participant data for research.

From the mobile application's point of view, the Bridge server handles the following activities:

- Establishing and verifying accounts
- Verifying a study participant's login credentials
- Collecting informed consent
- Collecting study data
- De-identifying the study's data using cryptographic techniques
- Maintaining separation between the participant's identity and their data
- Customizing surveys and schedules

Sage has a second cloud-based platform named Synapse. This informatics platform is a repository of tools and models that allow scientists to share and analyze data together in a visible and traceable manner. The structured data from the `Bridge` server will be fed to Synapse for storage and analysis by the research community

In *Chapter 8, Where to Go from Here* you will learn about the AppCore repository, a complementary repository to ResearchKit, that provides code to easily connect with the Sage Bridge REST API using their iOS SDK.

Note that there are other service providers available for backend services to ResearchKit-based apps. However, due to a lack of experience in using such services, we are not providing a list of such providers.

Introduction to sample ResearchKit backend server

In order to learn how to serialize task results to upload to backend services, let's use a simple backend server that's available as part of the Softwareitis project, called RKBackendServerSample. You can find the files corresponding to this chapter in the Chapter_7 folder of the RKBook.

The RKBackendServerSample folder contains a simple Ruby Sinatra-based open source backend server that accepts file uploads and stores the uploaded files in the ~/Desktop/RKBackendServerFiles folder. You can install Sinatra by typing the following command in the **Terminal** app (In some Macs, you may have to type sudo gem install sinatra):

```
gem install sinatra
```

Then you can start the server using the following:

```
cd <path to RKBackendServerSample folder>
ruby RKBackendServerSample.rb
```

In order to upload to the server, the task results need to be serialized first. In the next section, you will learn how to serialize ORKTaskResult objects.

Serialization of task results

You may recall from the previous chapters that the result of a finished task is available in the ORKTaskResult object from the result property of a task view controller. There are several ways to serialize this ORKTaskResult object. In this chapter, we will create a dictionary representation of the object, convert it to JSON using the NSJSONSerialization API, and create a ZIP archive of the JSON. This ZIP archive will then be uploaded to the backend server.

The serialization of survey responses

To present a survey and generate a survey result, let's add the following rows entry in the setupTableViewRows method of TableViewController.swift:

```
["Survey with Upload" : (didSelectMethod: self.showSurvey,
processResultMethod: self.processResultsWithUpload)]
```

The self.showSurvey method presents the same survey that we created in *Chapter 3, Building Surveys*. The self.processResultsWithUpload is a new method that needs to be added to process the result from the survey and upload it to the backend server.

Open the BackendUpload.swift file to follow along with the following code.

First, let's add the dictFromTaskResult method that converts a task result to a dictionary:

```
func dictFromTaskResult(taskResult: ORKTaskResult, zipArchive:
ZZArchive) -> [String : AnyObject]?
{
    var retDict : [String:AnyObject] = [:]
    //1
    retDict["taskRunUUID"] = taskResult.taskRunUUID.UUIDString
    retDict["startDate"] = "\(taskResult.startDate!)"
    retDict["endDate"] = "\(taskResult.endDate!)"
    //2
    for result in taskResult.results!
    {
        if let stepResult = result as? ORKStepResult
        {
            //3
            retDict[stepResult.identifier] =
dictFromStepResult(stepResult, zipArchive: zipArchive) ?? [:]
        }
    }
    //4
    return [taskResult.identifier : retDict]
}
```

Ignore the zipArchive parameter for now as we will cover it later in this chapter.

1. This stores taskRunUUID, start date, and end date
2. This loops through the step results inside a task result in a for loop
3. This uses the dictFromStepResult method to convert step results to a dictionary

4. This returns the generated dictionary enclosed in another dictionary with the task result's identifier as the key

Now let's look at the implementation of the `dictFromStepResult` method:

```
func dictFromStepResult(stepResult: ORKStepResult, zipArchive:
ZZArchive) -> [String : AnyObject]?
{
    var retDict : [String:AnyObject] = [:]
    //1
    retDict["startDate"] = "\(stepResult.startDate!)"
    retDict["endDate"] = "\(stepResult.endDate!)"
    //2
    for result in stepResult.results!
    {
        //3
        if result is ORKQuestionResult
        {
            //4
            retDict["\((result as! ORKQuestionResult).questionType.
stringValue())"] = "\((result as! ORKQuestionResult).stringValue())"
        }
    }
    return retDict
}
```

As mentioned above, ignore the `zipArchive` parameter for now.

1. This stores the start and end date of a step. This is useful to measure the amount of time that the participant spent on each step.

2. This loops through the results inside a step result in a `for` loop. Unless it's a form step, the step result usually contains only one result inside of a step result.

3. This checks whether the result is of the `ORKQuestionResult` type. All the survey responses will be of this type.

4. This uses the custom `stringValue` methods to convert `ORKQuestionType` enum and `ORKQuestionResult` to a string.

The `stringValue` is added as an extension to `ORKQuestionType` enum as follows. This method uses a simple switch statement to convert the enum value to a string:

```
extension ORKQuestionType
{
    func stringValue() -> String
    {
```

```
            var retString = "None"
            switch self
            {
            case .None:
                retString = "None"
            case .Scale:
                retString = "Scale"
            case .SingleChoice:
                retString = "SingleChoice"
            case .MultipleChoice:
                retString = "MultipleChoice"
            case .Decimal:
                retString = "Integer"
            case .Integer:
                retString = "Integer"
            case .Boolean:
                retString = "Boolean"
            case .Eligibility:
                retString = "Eligibility"
            case .Text:
                retString = "Text"
            case .TimeOfDay:
                retString = "TimeOfDay"
            case .DateAndTime:
                retString = "DateAndTime"
            case .Date:
                retString = "Date"
            case .TimeInterval:
                retString = "TimeInterval"
            case .Location:
                retString = "Location"
            }
            return retString
        }
    }
```

The stringValue method of ORKQuestionResult is shown in the following code. This method accesses the appropriate answer property of ORKQuestionResult depending on the type of question and converts the answer to string using the description property:

```
extension ORKQuestionResult
{
    func stringValue() ->String
    {
        var retString = "None"
        switch self.questionType
```

```
        {
        case .None:
            retString = "None"
        case .Scale:
            retString = (self as! ORKScaleQuestionResult).
scaleAnswer?.description ?? "Skipped"
        case .SingleChoice:
            fallthrough
        case .MultipleChoice:
            retString = (self as! ORKChoiceQuestionResult).
choiceAnswers?.description ?? "Skipped"
        case .Decimal:
            fallthrough
        case .Integer:
            retString = (self as! ORKNumericQuestionResult).
numericAnswer?.description ?? "Skipped"
        case .Boolean:
            fallthrough
        case .Eligibility:
            retString = (self as! ORKBooleanQuestionResult).
booleanAnswer?.description ?? "Skipped"
        case .Text:
            retString = (self as! ORKTextQuestionResult).textAnswer ??
"Skipped"
        case .TimeOfDay:
            retString = (self as! ORKTimeOfDayQuestionResult).
dateComponentsAnswer?.description ?? "Skipped"
        case .DateAndTime:
            fallthrough
        case .Date:
            retString = (self as! ORKDateQuestionResult).dateAnswer?.
description ?? "Skipped"
        case .TimeInterval:
            retString = (self as! ORKTimeIntervalQuestionResult).
intervalAnswer?.description ?? "Skipped"
        case .Location:
            retString = (self as! ORKLocationQuestionResult).
locationAnswer?.description ?? "Skipped"
        }
        return retString
    }
}
```

With the help of the preceding methods, we can now implement the processResultsWithUpload method to process the survey result and upload to the server, as shown in the following code:

```
func processResultsWithUpload(taskResult: ORKTaskResult?)
{
    do
    {
        //1
        let path = try createUniqueTaskResultsFolder(taskResult!.
taskRunUUID)
        let zipPath = (path as NSString).
stringByAppendingPathComponent("\(taskResult!.taskRunUUID.UUIDString).
zip")
        let zipArchive = try ZZArchive(URL: NSURL(fileURLWithPath:
zipPath), options: [ZZOpenOptionsCreateIfMissingKey : true])

        //2
        if let dict = dictFromTaskResult(taskResult!, zipArchive:
zipArchive) where NSJSONSerialization.isValidJSONObject(dict)
        {
            //3
            let json = try NSJSONSerialization.
dataWithJSONObject(dict, options: .PrettyPrinted)
            print(String(data: json, encoding: NSUTF8StringEncoding)!)
            //4
            try writeToZip(zipArchive, data: json, fileName:
"taskResult.json")
            //5
            uploadZipToRKBackendServer(zipPath)
        }
        else
        {
            print("Cannot convert to JSON")
        }
    }
    catch
    {
        print(error)
    }
}
```

1. This creates a unique folder and ZIP archive to store the task result files. To create ZIP archives, we will be using a third-party open source library called zipzap.

2. This calls the `dictFromTaskResult` method that we just created. It also checks whether the dictionary can be converted to JSON.

3. This converts the dictionary to a JSON object and prints it in the console.

4. This writes the JSON object to the ZIP archive as a `taskResult.json` file.

5. This uploads the ZIP file to `RKBackendServerSample`.

> **Note:** Apple strongly recommends that you encrypt the data sent to the backend service using **Cryptographic Message Syntax** (**CMS**) or similar encryption techniques. In *Chapter 8, Where to Go from Here* you will learn how to use the OpenSSL library to create a CMS envelope for the data.

The `uploadZipToRKBackendServer` method is implemented as follows:

```
func uploadZipToRKBackendServer(path: String)
{
    let data: NSData = NSData(contentsOfFile: path)!
    //1
    let RKBackendServerURL = "http://localhost:4567/upload/\((path as
NSString).lastPathComponent)"
    //2
    let request = NSMutableURLRequest(URL: NSURL(string:
RKBackendServerURL)!)
    request.HTTPMethod = "POST"
    request.setValue("Keep-Alive", forHTTPHeaderField: "Connection")
    request.setValue("application/zip", forHTTPHeaderField: "Content-
Type")
    //3
    let task = NSURLSession.sharedSession().
uploadTaskWithRequest(request, fromData: data) { (_, response, error)
-> Void in
        if error == nil && (response! as! NSHTTPURLResponse).
statusCode == 200
        {
            print("Successfully uploaded task results!")
        }
        else
        {
            print(error)
        }
    }
    task.resume()
}
```

The explanation of the above code is given as below:

1. Localhost is used as the server address in `RKBackendServerURL`, which assumes that the app is run in the Xcode simulator. Change this to your Mac's IP address to run it in an iOS device.

2. This creates `NSURLRequest` to upload the ZIP file.

3. This uses the `uploadTaskWithRequest` method of `NSURLSession` to upload. Note that this implementation ignores all the complexities of networking. In the production environment, you are highly encouraged to follow the guidelines provided by Apple in the *Networking Overview* document.

Once the app is executed and survey is answered, it will print the JSON result as follows:

```
{
  "first survey" : {
    "question 1" : {
      "startDate" : "2015-11-28 17:23:12 +0000",
      "Boolean" : "1",
      "endDate" : "2015-11-28 17:23:14 +0000"
    },
    "Completion Step" : {
      "startDate" : "2015-11-28 17:23:22 +0000",
      "endDate" : "2015-11-28 17:23:24 +0000"
    },
    "question 2" : {
      "startDate" : "2015-11-28 17:23:14 +0000",
      "Integer" : "Skipped",
      "endDate" : "2015-11-28 17:23:16 +0000"
    },
    "taskRunUUID" : "A51C87C5-64D5-4F12-90A4-EC3AE1EF3243",
    "Instruction Step" : {
      "startDate" : "2015-11-28 17:23:11 +0000",
      "endDate" : "2015-11-28 17:23:12 +0000"
    },
    "endDate" : "2015-11-28 17:23:24 +0000",
    "question 5" : {
      "startDate" : "2015-11-28 17:23:20 +0000",
      "Date" : "2015-11-28 17:23:20 +0000",
      "endDate" : "2015-11-28 17:23:21 +0000"
    },
    "startDate" : "2015-11-28 17:23:11 +0000",
    "question 3" : {
```

```
        "startDate" : "2015-11-28 17:23:16 +0000",
        "Scale" : "5",
        "endDate" : "2015-11-28 17:23:18 +0000"
      },
      "question 4" : {
        "startDate" : "2015-11-28 17:23:18 +0000",
        "SingleChoice" : "[1]",
        "endDate" : "2015-11-28 17:23:20 +0000"
      },
      "question 6" : {
        "startDate" : "2015-11-28 17:23:21 +0000",
        "TimeInterval" : "60",
        "endDate" : "2015-11-28 17:23:22 +0000"
      }
    }
  }
}
```

Serialization of file results

In the preceding section, you learned how to serialize survey responses. Now, let's learn about serializing results from other types of tasks. Specifically, let's look at a task that produces ORKFileResult such as the sustained phonation task that you learned in *Chapter 5, Active Tasks*.

To present a sustained phonation task and generate a result, let's add the following rows entry in the setupTableViewRows method of TableViewController.swift:

```
["Sustained Phonation with Upload" : (didSelectMethod: self.
showSustainedPhonationTask, processResultMethod: self.
processResultsWithUpload)]
```

The self.showSustainedPhonationTask method presents the sustained phonation task that we created in Chapter 5. We can reuse the preceding self.processResultsWithUpload method as it already provides you with a common infrastructure to handle all types of results.

The only addition that is needed is to the dictFromStepResult method. Add the following else if condition to this method:

```
            //1
            else if result is ORKFileResult
            {
                let fileResult = result as! ORKFileResult
                //2
                retDict["contentType"] = fileResult.contentType ??
"Unknown Type"
```

```
                    //3
                    if let filePath = fileResult.fileURL?.path
                    {
                        do
                        {
                            //4
                            try writeToZip(zipArchive, path: filePath)
                        }
                        catch
                        {
                            print(error)
                        }
                        //5
                        retDict["filePath"] = (filePath as NSString).
lastPathComponent
                    }
                }
```

The explanation of the above code is given below:

1. This checks whether `result` is of the `ORKFileResult` type.
2. This sets the content type of the return dictionary from the file result.
3. This reads the path of the file from `fileURL` of the file result.
4. This writes the audio file to the ZIP archive. The `zipArchive` parameter in `dictFromTaskResult` and `dictFromStepResult` methods comes in handy.
5. This stores the filename in the `filePath` key in the return dictionary. This key could indicate to the backend service to look for a file with the same name inside the ZIP archive.

Once the app is executed and phonation task is completed, it will print the JSON result and the ZIP archive will contain the two audio files referred in the JSON object:

```
{
  "SustainedPhonationTask" : {
    "conclusion" : {
      "startDate" : "2015-11-28 17:54:26 +0000",
      "endDate" : "2015-11-28 17:54:28 +0000"
    },
    "countdown" : {
      "startDate" : "2015-11-28 17:54:05 +0000",
      "contentType" : "audio\/m4a",
      "filePath" : "audio_B84F7DFE-A2E4-41C0-815D-C442A19DB824.m4a",
      "endDate" : "2015-11-28 17:54:11 +0000"
    },
```

```
     "taskRunUUID" : "B0FD6DB6-16C2-4711-A035-01D8F09E0EFB",
     "endDate" : "2015-11-28 17:54:28 +0000",      "audio" : {
        "startDate" : "2015-11-28 17:54:11 +0000",        "contentType" :
 "audio m4a",
        "filePath" : "audio_1C37B47D-A2DB-46E5-9BDB-CD837D0BE6A7.m4a",
        "endDate" : "2015-11-28 17:54:26 +0000"
     },
     "startDate" : "2015-11-28 17:54:03 +0000",
     "instruction" : {
        "startDate" : "2015-11-28 17:54:03 +0000",
        "endDate" : "2015-11-28 17:54:04 +0000"
     },
     "instruction1" : {
        "startDate" : "2015-11-28 17:54:04 +0000",
        "endDate" : "2015-11-28 17:54:05 +0000"
     }
   }
 }
}
```

Using a similar technique, results from other types of active and consent tasks can be serialized. The results that cannot be converted to a dictionary can be stored as a file in the ZIP archive and the JSON object can provide references to the stored files.

Summary

In this chapter, you learned ways to serialize task results and upload the results to a simple backend server. We also discussed Sage and its `Bridge` service. The next chapter will provide you with a lot of information about tools and techniques to use in your real-world ResearchKit application.

8
Where to Go from Here

This chapter covers miscellaneous topics related to the development of a ResearchKit-based application. This includes task restoration, presenting graphs and charts, scheduling, safeguarding data using OpenSSL, and a theoretical architecture for ResearchKit applications. Additionally, online resource, including references to source code and other development items, are identified.

Restoring tasks

In clinical research studies, surveys may get lengthy and take a long time to complete. Also, in many cases, the users might have to find the information being asked from other places such as paper medical records, and so on. In these cases, it would be convenient if the users can save the partially completed survey and resume it later. ResearchKit provides a mechanism to save the partially completed surveys through the restorationData property and other delegate methods in ORKTaskViewController. Let's learn how to add a restorable survey in detail in this chapter.

In the following sections, we will be adding Restorable Survey to the lists of tasks in the Softwareitis project.

First, let's add the showRestorableSurvey method in RestorableSurvey. swift. This method replicates the survey created in *Chapter 3, Building Surveys* as showSurvey with one difference: The identifier of the survey task is set to "Restorable Survey", as shown in the following:

```
func showRestorableSurvey()
{
  // ...
  // question steps creation from showSurvey method of Chapter 3 goes
  here
```

```
// ....

    let task = ORKOrderedTask(identifier: "Restorable Survey", steps:
[instStep, question1, question2, question3, question4, question5,
question6, completionStep])
    let taskViewController = ORKTaskViewController(task: task,
taskRunUUID: nil)
    taskViewController.delegate = self
    presentViewController(taskViewController, animated: true,
completion: nil)
}
```

Then, let's add this task to the list of tasks in `TableViewController` by adding the following row to the `taskRows` array in the `setupTableViewRows` method:

```
["Restorable Survey" : (didSelectMethod: self.showRestorableSurvey,
processResultMethod: self.processRestorableSurveyResults)]
```

The above code adds a new `Restorable Survey` row in the tasks list. However, this survey is not restorable yet. Let's perform the following three steps to make this survey restorable:

Implement the `taskViewControllerSupportsSaveAndRestore` `(taskViewController: ORKTaskViewController)` delegate method of `ORKTaskViewControllerDelegate` in `TableViewController.swift` to return `true` if the identifier of task of the task view controller is `Restorable Survey`, as follows:

```
func taskViewControllerSupportsSaveAndRestore(taskViewController:
ORKTaskViewController) -> Bool {
    return taskViewController.task?.identifier ==
restorableSurveyIdentifier
}
```

Create two properties, `savedRestorationData` and `savedTask`, in `TableViewController` to save the restoration data and task in memory. Restoration data is an opaque `NSData` object that represents the partially answered survey. Modify the `taskViewController(taskViewController: ORKTaskViewController, didFinishWithReason reason: ORKTaskViewControllerFinishReason, error: NSError?)` delegate method to check for `ORKTaskViewControllerFinishReason.Saved`, as shown in the following:

```
func taskViewController(taskViewController: ORKTaskViewController,
didFinishWithReason reason: ORKTaskViewControllerFinishReason, error:
NSError?)
{
    //Resets the properties
    savedTask = nil
    savedRestorationData = nil
```

```
        if reason == .Completed
        {
            if let indexPath = tappedIndexPath
            {
                let rowDict = taskRows[indexPath.row]
                if let tuple = rowDict.values.first
                {
                    tuple.processResultMethod(taskViewController.result)
                }
            }
        }
        else if reason == .Saved
        {
            //1
            savedTask = taskViewController.task
            savedRestorationData = taskViewController.restorationData
        }
        dismissViewControllerAnimated(true, completion: nil)
    }
```

If `ORKTaskViewControllerFinishReason` is `Saved`, then save `restorationData` and `task` from `taskViewController` in the properties that we created earlier. Note that you can also choose to store the restoration data and task in the filesystem using the `writeToFile` method of `NSData` and `NSKeyedArchiver`.

Modify the `tableView(tableView: UITableView, didSelectRowAtIndexPath indexPath: NSIndexPath)` method in `TableViewController` to check whether there is already saved data, as shown in the following:

```
override func tableView(tableView: UITableView,
didSelectRowAtIndexPath indexPath: NSIndexPath) {
    tableView.deselectRowAtIndexPath(indexPath, animated: true)
    if  indexPath.section == taskRowSection && indexPath.row ==
restorableSurveyRow && savedRestorationData != nil && savedTask != nil
    {
        //1
        let taskViewController = ORKTaskViewController(task:
savedTask!, restorationData: savedRestorationData!, delegate: self)
        presentViewController(taskViewController, animated: true,
completion: nil)
    }
    else
    {
        // ...
        //process normally
        // ...
    }
}
```

If there is data in the `savedRestorationData` and `savedTask` properties, we will invoke the `ORKTaskViewController(task: ORKTask?, restorationData data: NSData?, delegate: ORKTaskViewControllerDelegate?)` initializer to recreate task view controller with the saved data.

Using the preceding three steps, we added the save and restore functionality to the `Restorable Survey` task. To test this functionality, start the survey, answer a few questions, and press the **Cancel** button. You will be presented a menu similar to the following screenshot:

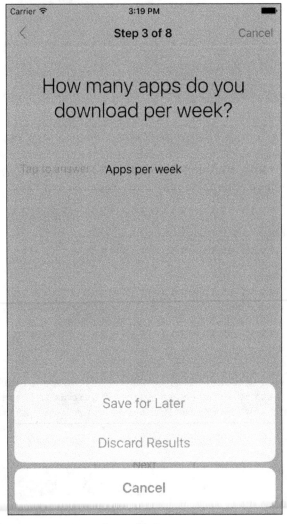

Restorable Survey

Pressing **Save for Later** saves the current progress. When the restorable survey is launched again, you will notice that the survey resumes from where it was saved.

Graphs and charts

In clinical research apps, it is useful to show the summary of the users' task results and other pertinent health information in the form of a dashboard. Dashboards can improve the user engagement and be a tool in helping the users manage their condition. Using graphs and charts, the dashboards can be easily created. Out of the box, ResearchKit already comes with easy-to-use graphs. In this section, let's study how to use ORKPieChartView, ORKLineGraphChartView, and ORKDiscreteGraphChartView to create charts and graphs.

The GraphTableViewController contains a static table view with three table view cells, each containing one type of graph or chart view. Also, Graphs Scene in the Main.storyboard file shows the UI for GraphTableViewController.

Pie chart

The ORKPieChartView, a sub class of UIView, helps in creating a pie chart. It requires a dataSource object that implements the ORKPieChartViewDataSource protocol. The GraphTableViewController implements this protocol as shown in the following:

```
extension GraphTableViewController : ORKPieChartViewDataSource
{
    //1
    func numberOfSegmentsInPieChartView(pieChartView: ORKPieChartView)
-> Int {
        return 3
    }
    //2
    func pieChartView(pieChartView: ORKPieChartView,
valueForSegmentAtIndex index: Int) -> CGFloat {
        return 33
    }
    //3
    func pieChartView(pieChartView: ORKPieChartView,
colorForSegmentAtIndex index: Int) -> UIColor {
        let colors = [UIColor.blueColor(), UIColor.redColor(),
UIColor.purpleColor()]
        return colors[index]
```

```
//4
    func pieChartView(pieChartView: ORKPieChartView,
titleForSegmentAtIndex index: Int) -> String {
        return "Segment \(index+1)"
    }
}
```

The explanation of the above code is given as below:

- Returns the number of segments needed in the pie chart.
- Returns the value for each segment (hard coded to 33). In your app, return the appropriate value for each segment.
- Returns the color for each segment.
- Returns the title for each segment.
- Refer to the ORKPieChartView documentation for further customization options.

Line graph

The ORKLineGraphChartView, a sub class of ORKGraphChartView, helps in creating a line graph. It requires a dataSource object that implements the ORKGraphChartViewDataSource protocol. Each point in the line graph is represented by the ORKRangedPoint object. We will be plotting the following points on the graph. Note the absence of data is shown with ORKRangedPoint(), as follows:

```
let linePlotPoints =
[

    ORKRangedPoint(value: 10),
    ORKRangedPoint(value: 20),
    ORKRangedPoint(value: 25),
    ORKRangedPoint(),
    ORKRangedPoint(value: 30),
    ORKRangedPoint(value: 40),

]
```

The ORKGraphChartViewDataSource is implemented as shown below:

```
extension GraphTableViewController : ORKGraphChartViewDataSource
{
    //1
    func numberOfPlotsInGraphChartView(graphChartView:
ORKGraphChartView) -> Int {
```

```
        return 1
    }
    //2
    func graphChartView(graphChartView: ORKGraphChartView,
numberOfPointsForPlotIndex plotIndex: Int) -> Int {
        return 6
    }
    //3
    func graphChartView(graphChartView: ORKGraphChartView,
pointForPointIndex pointIndex: Int, plotIndex: Int) -> ORKRangedPoint
{
        return graphChartView is ORKLineGraphChartView ?
linePlotPoints[pointIndex] : discretePlotPoints[pointIndex]
    }
    //4
    func graphChartView(graphChartView: ORKGraphChartView,
colorForPlotIndex plotIndex: Int) -> UIColor {
        return UIColor.purpleColor()
    }
    //5
    func maximumValueForGraphChartView(graphChartView:
ORKGraphChartView) -> CGFloat {
        return 70
    }
    //6
    func minimumValueForGraphChartView(graphChartView:
ORKGraphChartView) -> CGFloat {
        return 0
    }
    //7
    func graphChartView(graphChartView: ORKGraphChartView,
titleForXAxisAtPointIndex pointIndex: Int) -> String? {
        return "\(pointIndex + 1)"
    }
}
```

The explanation of the above code is given as below:

- Returns the number of plots in the line graph (hard coded to 1 for simplicity).
- Returns the number of points in the plot (hard coded to 6 for simplicity).
- Returns the ORKRangedPoint object from the linePlotPoints array. Ignore discretePlotPoints for now.
- Returns the color for the plot point.

- Returns the maximum value for the graph, this is needed to adjust the *y* axis.

- Returns the minimum value for the graph this is needed to adjust the *y* axis.

- Returns the title for points in *x* axis.

- Refer to the ORKLineGraphChartView documentation for further customization options.

Discrete graph

The ORKDiscreteGraphChartView, a sub class of ORKGraphChartView, helps in creating a discrete graph. It requires a dataSource object that implements the ORKGraphChartViewDataSource protocol. Similar to the line graph, each point in the discrete graph is represented by the ORKRangedPoint object. We will be plotting the following points on the graph. Note that discrete graph can take ranges instead of just points. You can specify a range using the ORKRangedPoint (minumumValue:maximumValue) initializer, as follows:

```
let discretePlotPoints =
[
    ORKRangedPoint(minimumValue: 10, maximumValue: 18),
    ORKRangedPoint(value: 15),
    ORKRangedPoint(value: 20),
    ORKRangedPoint(minimumValue: 25, maximumValue: 30),
    ORKRangedPoint(minimumValue: 32, maximumValue: 38),
    ORKRangedPoint(minimumValue: 40, maximumValue: 48),
]
```

This graph uses the same delegate methods as the line graph. Therefore, we can reuse the code from the previous section.

Refer to the ORKDiscreteGraphChartView documentation for further customization options.

The following image shows the screenshot of all the three graphs:

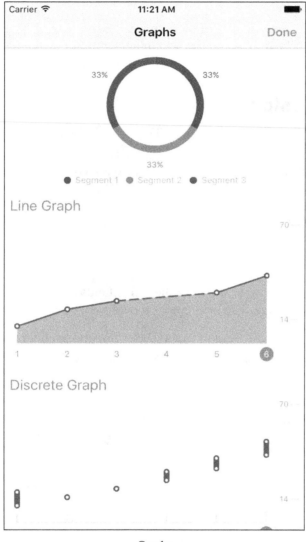

Graphs

Scheduling

The five initial ResearchKit-based applications asked the participants to perform tasks on a periodic basis. The recurring nature of these tasks are controlled by schedules embedded in the application or retrieved from the server. The ability to retrieve the schedules from the server allows the researchers to modify when the tasks are presented to the participants and, if necessary, prevent the task from being presented.

The ability to schedule periodic presentation of tasks to the participant is controlled by a schedule expression. Schedule expressions are backed by cron expressions, a scheduling concept that originated in Unix-like operating systems. Using cron expressions, an infinite sequence of moments can be expressed. These moments may then correspond to the time when the researchers would like the participants to carry out a task.

Cron expressions

Cron expressions are strings and they support recurrence pattern based on the following:

- The day of the week (Sunday, Monday, and so on)
- Month (January, February, and so on)
- Day of the month (1-31)
- Hours (0-23)
- Minutes (0-59)

A cron expression is a concatenation of these five fields, where the fields are separated by white spaces. The value in each field may be one of the following:

- An "*". For example, an "*" in the Day of the month field means every day.
- An exact values. For example, a 1 in the Day of the week fields means every Monday.
- A list of value. For example, 7, 14, 21" for the Day of the month field means the 7th, 14th, and 21st day of the month.
- A range. For example, 9-12 for the month field means September to December.

A schedule is considered satisfied if all the date and time fields match the provided date and time, a logical conjunction. There is a partial relaxation if the day of the week and the day of the month are restricted (i.e., not *); these fields are a logical disjunction.

APCSchedule Expression

The AppCore framework provides supports for schedule with the APCScheduleExpression and APCScheduleEnumerator classes. The APCScheduleExpression class consumes a cron expression and returns an enumerator (instances of APCScheduleEnumerator) that allows applications to enumerate through date-time moments that satisfy the cron expression.

How to use the `APCScheduleExpression` is depicted in the following code block:

```
func exampleScheduleExpression()
{
    let dateFormatter = NSDateFormatter()
    dateFormatter.dateFormat = "yyyy-MM-dd HH:mm"
    let schedule      = APCScheduleExpression(expression: "5 10 15
2,4,6 *")
    let startDate     = dateFormatter.dateFromString("2015-01-01
06:00")
    let endDate       = dateFormatter.dateFromString("2016-01-01
06:00")
    let enumerator    = schedule.enumeratorBeginningAtTime(startDate,
endingAtTime: endDate)
    var date = enumerator.nextMoment()
    while date != nil
    {
        print(date)
        date = enumerator.nextMoment()
    }
}
```

The output from the preceding `exampleScheduleExpression` function is as follows:

2015-02-15 18:05:00 +0000

2015-04-15 17:05:00 +0000

2015-06-15 17:05:00 +0000

The `APCScheduleExpression` and supporting class form a utility-like component that is not dependent on other components in AppCore. As such, it may be an extract from AppCore and reused. For the reader's benefit, the source for the `APCScheduleExpression` has been included in the Softwareitis project.

Safeguarding Data-in-transit

The information collected by ResearchKit-based applications is likely to be considered sensitive information. It's only prudent that an application takes steps to safeguard the information while at rest and in transit. The initial ResearchKit applications employed OpenSSL to encrypt the data prior to uploading it to the server.

The initial ResearchKit applications used `NSURLSession` to upload the data in the background; the uploading was performed by the operating system. Given the security model used by iOS, the operating system would not have access to the data unless it was written to an unprotected area of the filesystem (that is, `NSFileProtectionNone`). Therefore, the data written to this area must be safeguarded cryptographically.

The specific OpenSSL feature used to safeguard the collected information was its **Cryptographic Message Syntax (CMS)** capability. Using the server's X509 certificate, the initial ResearchKit application CMS wrapped (that is, encrypts) the data so that only the holder of the private key associated with the certificate will be able to decrypt the data. The wrapping was performed prior to storing the data in an unprotected area of the filesystem on a device.

All the source code provided in this book is written in Swift. OpenSSL, however, is writing in the C programming language. While it is possible to invoke OpenSSL functions from Swift, the plethora of C-based macros will make the use of some OpenSSL functions and types challenging to use from Swift. Therefore, in the following listing, you'll find a C function implementation that encrypts provided data using CMS:

```c
NSData* cmsEncrypt(NSData* data, NSString* identityPath, NSError*
__autoreleasing* error)
{
    NSData* returnValue = nil;
    int     ret = 1;    //  Default to failed
    //  On OpenSSL 1.0.0 and later only: for streaming set CMS_STREAM
    int flags = CMS_STREAM | CMS_BINARY;
    OpenSSL_add_all_algorithms();
    ERR_load_crypto_strings();
    //  Read in recipient certificate
    BIO*    tbio = BIO_new_file([identityPath UTF8String], "r");
    if (!tbio)
        goto err;
    X509*   rcert = PEM_read_bio_X509(tbio, NULL, 0, NULL);
    if (!rcert)
        goto err;
    //  Create recipient STACK and add recipient cert to it
    STACK_OF(X509)* recips = sk_X509_new_null();
    if (!recips || !sk_X509_push(recips, rcert))
        goto err;
    //  sk_X509_pop_free will free up recipient STACK and
    //  its contents so set rcert to NULL so it isn't freed up twice.
    rcert = NULL;
    //  Open content being encrypted
    BIO*    in = BIO_new_mem_buf((void *)[data bytes], (int)[data
length]);
    if (!in)
        goto err;
    //  encrypt content
    CMS_ContentInfo*    cms = CMS_encrypt(recips, in, EVP_aes_128_
cbc(), flags);
```

```
    if (!cms)
        goto err;
    BIO*    out = BIO_new(BIO_s_mem());
    if (!out)
        goto err;
    // Stream the encrypted data into the buffer as DER
    if (!i2d_CMS_bio_stream(out, cms, in, flags))
        goto err;
    // Success
    ret = 0;
    // Convert the data
    BUF_MEM*    bptr = NULL;
    BIO_get_mem_ptr(out, &bptr);
    returnValue = [NSData dataWithBytes:bptr->data length:bptr-
>length];
err:
    if (ret)
    {
        if (error)
            *error = [NSError errorWithDomain:@"openssl" code:ret
userInfo:nil];
        fprintf(stderr, "Error Encrypting Data\n");
        ERR_print_errors_fp(stderr);
    }
    if (cms)
        CMS_ContentInfo_free(cms);
    if (rcert)
        X509_free(rcert);
    if (recips)
        sk_X509_pop_free(recips, X509_free);
    if (in)
        BIO_free(in);
    if (out)
        BIO_free(out);
    if (tbio)
        BIO_free(tbio);
    return returnValue;
}
```

In order to invoke the about cmsEncrypt function, an X509 certificate is required. For testing, you can generate a self-signed certificate using OpenSSL's command-line interface. Note that the generated private key is stored in key.pem and it is not password protected:

```
openssl req -x509 -newkey rsa:2048 -keyout key.pem -out cert.pem -days
1080 -nodes
```

The self-signed certificate will be generated by the preceding command and stored in the cert.pem file. For the application to use the certificate, it must be copied in the Xcode project and added to the "Copy Bundle Resources" phase under the "Build Phases" setting for the desired targets.

With the certificate in the application bundle, you can invoke the cmsEncrypt C function using Swift:

```
let plainText  = "Feed me chocolates".dataUsingEncoding(NSUTF8StringE
ncoding)
let certPath   = NSBundle.mainBundle().pathForResource("cert", ofType:
"pem")
let cipherText = cmsEncrypt(plainText, certPath, nil)
NSLog("%@", cipherText)
```

A theoretical architecture for ResearchKit-based applications

This section presents a generic architecture for a ResearchKit-based application that performs similar functions to the initial five applications that were released by Apple, as follows:

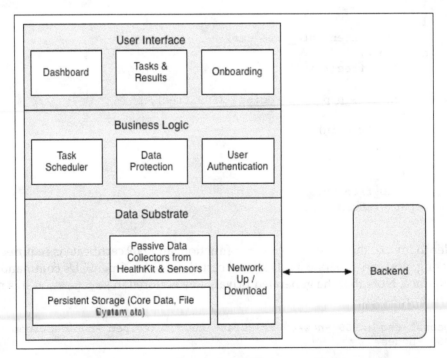

Generic Architecture

The presented architecture employs a layered approach in order to allocate responsibilities of the application. This provides for a clear separation of responsibilities, exposes the work flow, and the reduction of dependencies allows the layers to be replaced with minimum effort. This architecture attempts to minimize coupling between components, while maximizing cohesiveness of these components.

This layered architecture does not preclude the use of the **Model View Controller** (**MVC**) design pattern. The MVC design pattern integrates well with the layer architecture in that the various MVC comments will live in the different layers and they depend on lower layers for specific functionality.

Presentation layer

The presentation layer is responsible to create and display the user interface as well as handle the user interaction. This layer is dependent on and driven by the business logic layer.

The typical features with components that reside in the presentation layer are as follows:

- The presentation of the onboarding process
- The dashboard, where the tasks to be performed by the participant are listed
- Specific tasks: the visual components of each step in the tasks
- Task results

The first thing a new study participant will see when they launch a ResearchKit-based application is the presentation of the onboarding process. This process could consist of a study overview, performing an electronic consent, collecting login credentials for any backend services, and potentially presenting a comprehension quiz.

The dashboard component presents the list of tasks that the researcher would like the participant to perform that day or for some given period of time. This presentation should provide the level of effort and amount of time required of the participant for each given task. The dashboard could also present a summary in an icon form of the previous execution of the task.

The execution of tasks and collection of the resulting data is the heart and soul of a ResearchKit-based application. Therefore, most tasks will have some form of user interface in which the task will engage the participant. Whether it's presenting surveys, a fitness task, or a cognitive game, these tasks add to or use components in the presentation layer.

In order to keep the study participant engaged and increase the likelihood that they'll stay in the study, the application should present the results of the performed task. Ideally, the application should present the population norm along with the participant's results if it's necessary.

Business logic layer

The business logic layer encapsulates the encoding for the real-world rules that determine how data is created, displayed, and stored either locally or on a server. This layer indirectly controls what the study participant will see and what they will be able to do with the application.

The typical components that may be found in a business logic layer are as follows:

- User authentication state machine
- Data protection enforcement
- Task scheduler

Given the nature of the data that may be stored by a ResearchKit application, it is imperative that such applications ensure that all use of the application is only by the study participant. This could take many forms including the following:

- Authenticating the user to the device using Touch ID
- Authenticating the user via username and password check
- Second factor authentication
- Verification code
- Idle timeout
- Session timeout

Given the potential statefulness of user authentication, asynchronous state transition, and the need for high reliability, a state machine would address the needs rather elegantly.

Applications that require the participant to carry out tasks on periodic basis will require the support of schedules and scheduler. The schedule would identify when a task is to be performed and the scheduler would decide which task should be presented to the participant for a particular point in time.

There are numerous ways in which a schedule may be expressed. Possible attributes for such expressions could include the following components:

- Epoch: A date-time value that forms the lower bounds of the sequence of the date-time values

- Recurrence pattern: A generator based on the cron expression or ISO 8601

- Recurrence offset or delay: An ISO 8601 duration that's applied to the output of the recurrence pattern

- Maximum duration: An ISO 8601 duration that, when added to the epoch, forms the upper bounds of the sequence of the date-time values

- Maximum sequence length: An upper bound on the number of items that will appear in the date-time sequence

Data substrate layer

At their core, ResearchKit-based applications are about data. These applications collect and present data from a variety of sources including, but not limited to, persistent storage on the device, sensor data, HealthKit, and data received from the network. Encapsulating data access in one component alleviates rest of the application from the mired of different APIs, concurrency strategies, and error handling.

The data aggregation provided by the Data substrate layer includes data from the following:

- **HealthKit**: The data written to HealthKit by the user, third-party applications, and heart beat received from the Bluetooth-equipped heart-beat detectors.

- **Sensors**: The data from the GPS, accelerometer, and gyroscope.

- **Passive data collector**: With the participant's permission, the collection of data in the background without explicit triggering by the study participant. For example, a person's degree of socialization may be determined by looking at the relative distance traveled each day.

- **Data uploading and downloading**: The application may wish to download new schedules, surveys, and other data that directs the behavior of tasks. Additionally, the secure uploading of collected data could be supported by this component.

- **Persistent storage**: A result summary of the previous tasks performed as well as population averages could be stored in the filesystem for later retrieval by higher layers in the architecture.

Online ResearchKit resource

Apple open sourced ResearchKit and, as a result, the evolution of this framework is conducted on the Internet at `http://researchkit.org`. Additionally, numerous resources are available online including the following:

- ResearchKit source code on GitHub: `https://github.com/researchkit/researchkit`

- ResearchKit documentation: `http://researchkit.org/docs/docs/Overview/GuideOverview.html`

- ResearchKit developer's forum: `https://forums.developer.apple.com/community/researchkit`

- ResearchKit-Users: `https://lists.apple.com/mailman/listinfo/researchkit-users`

- ResearchKit-dev: `https://lists.apple.com/mailman/listinfo/researchkit-dev`

Each of the initial five ResearchKit-based applications were open sourced by Apple. The source code for these applications, including the common `AppCore` framework, resides on GitHub. The repositories for these applications are as follows:

- **MyHeart Counts**: Developed by Stanford University to study cardiovascular health: `https://github.com/ResearchKit/MyHeartCounts`

- **Share the Journey**: Developed by Sage Bionetworks to study breast cancer: `https://github.com/ResearchKit/ShareTheJourney`

- **mPower**: Developed by Sage Bionetworks and the University of Rochester to study Parkinson's disease: `https://github.com/ResearchKit/mPower`

- **Asthma Health**: Developed by Mount Sinai to study asthma: `https://github.com/ResearchKit/AsthmaHealth`

- **GlucoSuccess**: developed by Massachusetts General Hospital to study diabetes: `https://github.com/ResearchKit/GlucoSuccess`

- **AppCore**: Common code shared by all five applications: `https://github.com/ResearchKit/AppCore`

Summary

This chapter covered miscellaneous topics that are useful for many real-world ResearchKit applications. Also, we reviewed a theoretical architecture for ResearchKit-based applications. This chapter concludes this book. Hope you enjoyed reading this book as much as we, the authors, enjoyed writing it. We look forward to seeing many impressive ResearchKit-based applications that help the researchers get invaluable insights for diseases and help the patients manage their conditions better.

Index

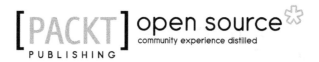

Thank you for buying
Getting Started with ResearchKit

About Packt Publishing

Packt, pronounced 'packed', published its first book, *Mastering phpMyAdmin for Effective MySQL Management*, in April 2004, and subsequently continued to specialize in publishing highly focused books on specific technologies and solutions.

Our books and publications share the experiences of your fellow IT professionals in adapting and customizing today's systems, applications, and frameworks. Our solution-based books give you the knowledge and power to customize the software and technologies you're using to get the job done. Packt books are more specific and less general than the IT books you have seen in the past. Our unique business model allows us to bring you more focused information, giving you more of what you need to know, and less of what you don't.

Packt is a modern yet unique publishing company that focuses on producing quality, cutting-edge books for communities of developers, administrators, and newbies alike. For more information, please visit our website at www.packtpub.com.

About Packt Open Source

In 2010, Packt launched two new brands, Packt Open Source and Packt Enterprise, in order to continue its focus on specialization. This book is part of the Packt Open Source brand, home to books published on software built around open source licenses, and offering information to anybody from advanced developers to budding web designers. The Open Source brand also runs Packt's Open Source Royalty Scheme, by which Packt gives a royalty to each open source project about whose software a book is sold.

Writing for Packt

We welcome all inquiries from people who are interested in authoring. Book proposals should be sent to author@packtpub.com. If your book idea is still at an early stage and you would like to discuss it first before writing a formal book proposal, then please contact us; one of our commissioning editors will get in touch with you.

We're not just looking for published authors; if you have strong technical skills but no writing experience, our experienced editors can help you develop a writing career, or simply get some additional reward for your expertise.

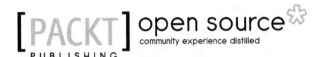

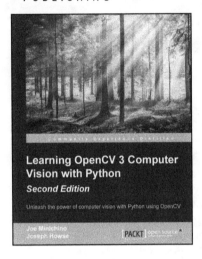

Learning OpenCV 3 Computer Vision with Python

Second Edition

ISBN: 978-1-78528-384-0   Paperback: 266 pages

Unleash the power of computer vision with Python using OpenCV

1. Create impressive applications with OpenCV and Python.

2. Familiarize yourself with advanced machine learning concepts.

3. Harness the power of computer vision with this easy-to-follow guide.

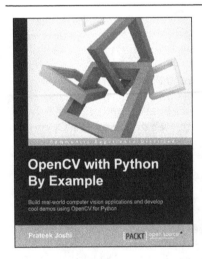

OpenCV with Python By Example

ISBN: 978-1-78528-393-2   Paperback: 296 pages

Build real-world computer vision applications and develop cool demos using OpenCV for Python

1. Learn how to apply complex visual effects to images using geometric transformations and image filters.

2. Extract features from an image and use them to develop advanced applications.

3. Build algorithms to understand the image content and recognize objects in an image.

Please check **www.PacktPub.com** for information on our titles

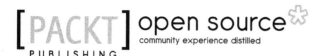

[PACKT] open source *
PUBLISHING   community experience distilled

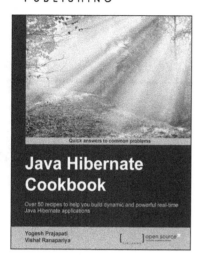

Java Hibernate Cookbook
ISBN: 978-1-78439-190-4   Paperback: 250 pages

Over 50 recipes to help you build dynamic and powerful real-time Java Hibernate applications

1. Learn to associate JDBC and Hibernate with object persistence.

2. Manage association mappings, implement basic annotations and learn caching.

3. Get to grips with Hibernate fundamentals from installation to developing a businessapplication with this step-by-step guide.

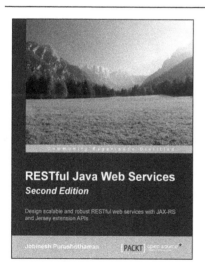

RESTful Java Web Services
Second Edition
ISBN: 978-1-78439-909-2   Paperback: 354 pages

Design scalable and robust RESTful web services with JAX-RS and Jersey extension APIs

1. Get to grips with the portable Java APIs used for JSON processing.

2. Design solutions to produce, consume, and visualize RESTful web services using WADL, RAML, and Swagger.

3. A step-by-step guide packed with many real-life use-cases to help you build efficient and secure RESTful web APIs in Java.

Please check **www.PacktPub.com** for information on our titles